DIY Cancer Repair Manual by Joseph & Sari Grove
including: DIY Diagnostic Imaging (see more at http://www.grovecanada.ca)

Table Of Contents

So you want to go "alternative" with your cancer treatment but you don't know where to start...

by Sari - Thursday, August 20, 2015

http://grovecanada.ca/so-you-want-to-go-alternative-with-your-cancer-treatment-but-you-dont-know-where-to-start/

So you want to go "alternative" with your cancer treatment but you don't know where to start...

I can help with that...

I will try & make this as simple as possible...

Below is my Grove Body Part Chart...

There are 12 "body parts" listed under the column "Organ"...(Gender refers to the Prostate gland in men, & in women it is called Skene's gland & sits in the same location...)

Each body part contains a MINUS element & a PLUS element...

Minus elements CLEAN the body part...

Plus elements FEED the body part...

Cancer is a disease of EXCESS, so it requires DETOX or CLEANING...

Ok, so...To keep it simple...A solid alternative anticancer protocol would be to simply choose the entire MINUS column...

Everything in the Minus column is a detoxer...

So you will be cleaning out each body part systematically...

What are the numbers?

Ok, so the numbers are how strong an element is…

The STRONGEST MINUS element is -12 Boron…

The strongest PLUS element is +12 Lead…

The elements in the Minus & Plus pile are opposites…

So if you raise one, you will also lower the other…Like a seesaw…

The elements on the chart are from the Periodic Table of elements…In the real world you will find these elements in real things with different names…After a while you will start to know which element is what in the real world & what it does & what its side effects are…It is handy to know this because there are so many words being thrown at you in alternative cancer treatment protocols, if you are able to figure out what things are on the Grove Body Part Chart, you will be able to simplify your own choices for a protocol…

Please Note:The elements to AVOID when detoxifying the body & brain from Cancer are ALL the PLUS elements…(Remember, EACH element represents a FAMILY of things in the real world…For example, Calcium is found in all dairy products, Coral, Chasteberry Vitex/Vitus Agnus Castus, & Vitamin K2…Calcium is a PLUS element, with a strength of +5, which means it is less strong than a potato at +12, but more strong than a Bean or Pulse like a Chickpea at +1…So when choosing your foods, understand that if you must eat PLUS elements, choose the weakest ones…A bean has less strength than a potato…So it will feed the parasites less…)

Grove Body Part Chart		
Organ	Minus -F Element	Plus +M Element
Thyroid	-1 Zinc	Lead +12
Thymus	Manganese -2	Iron +11
Lungs & Lymph Nodes	Titanium -3	Aluminum +10
Heart	-4 Potassium	Aurum +9
Kidneys	-5 Carbon	Nitrogen +8
Pancreas	-6 Selenium	Sugar +7
Liver	-7 Oxygen	Hydrogen +6
Adrenal Gland	Iodine -8	Calcium +5
Spleen	Copper -9	Phosphorus +4
Gallbladder	Magnesium -10	Mercury +3
Colon	-11 Fluorine	Bismuth +2
Gender F or M	Boron -12	Molybdenum +1

Corrected for Sugar

Ok, so I will give an example of a Minus protocol in real world words...(note: these are all families of things that live in the real world...Don't take these words literally...Zinc is just a catch all phrase for all those things like ginger root, vitamin C, vitamin D3, turmeric, sunshine etc....Each one represents a myriad of things in the real world...For simplicity, I group them into categories)...

You are looking for:

Zinc

Manganese

Titanium

Potassium

Carbon

Selenium

Oxygen

Iodine

Copper

Magnesium

Fluorine

Boron

These are all the MINUS elements…The cleansing elements…

Ok, so here are some examples:

Zinc: Vitamin D3 50,000 iu/week, Ginger root boiled tea, megadose Vitamin C, Camu Camu powder, Wormwood, fruit, Apple cider vinegar, sunshine, heat, saunas, steam, tanning beds(really- especially in winter climates)

Note:What got rid of my pneumonia

(probably caught from my husband, who caught it from a friend who had visited his dad in a hospital & probably picked up a Staphylococcus infection which is a LEAD excess on the Grove Body Part Chart-excess lead comes from old galvanized steel pipes degrading & losing their Zinc coating which brings them down to just Lead)

was 9 minutes in an intermediate level tanning bed(a Zinc on the Grove Body Part Chart) with their lotion on my whole front side…(cost about $25 total Canadian currency-at a tanning salon downstairs at Yonge & St. Clair in Toronto-North East corner basement of mall)

My husband's pneumonia responded to Cayenne Pepper(a Selenium on the Grove Body Part Chart) in everything he ate or drank...Like a giant teaspoon...(in soup, tea, coffee...) Another innovative Zinc family element:RubyLux 250 watt Infrared light bulb which can go into ANY light fixture-put it on your desk for while you are on the computer-shine it on your face to reduce swelling from dentistry, also helps to lower Lead levels in your whole body including those that cause toenail fungus...

Manganese:Bloodroot capsules, Mugwort herb,all Nuts, Pumpkin seeds , Manganese pills, ground Flaxseeds, Black walnut hull powder, Nutmeg, Flaxseed oil, sesame seeds, poppy seeds, homeopathic opium, Moxibustion, moxa, mugwort incense, Clove cigarettes, Nutmeg, Mugwort incense cones, Mugwort cigarettes, the Lily flower...

Titanium:CBD oil, *Frankincense essential oil(chew the resin & spit it out, or oral or topical), Mint leafs, Clove powder or Clove oil, Serrapeptase (has affinity for Lung & Lymph nodes as well as Cystic Fibrosis-also cleans Parietal lobe in brain)...Clove incense...Vanilla Beans- you can just chew them raw & swallow(about$3.49 Canadian currency for 2 at a grocery store, look behind the counter or ask(Dave Young grocery store at Eglinton near Bathurst has them)...(Mesenchymal cells feed on cholesterol which Titanium lowers)...

For brain tumours: Diffuse Frankincense oil in your room at night...(Sacred Frankincense from Young Living is one I know works)...Also rub on bottom of feet at night & at back of neck where head meets spine...(also diffuse, orange, lemon, clove, lavender at other times)...

*You can put a few drops in some water, or some coconut water, or some aloe juice...You can also buy Frankincense resin(the yellow bits) & chew them until they lose flavour then spit it out-that is how they do it in Oman(no cancer in Oman!)-it's cheaper when you chew it actually-I know the oil is expensive...sigh...But cheaper than CBD oil which acts in a similar fashion...You can also buy Boswellia pills as a supplement & that is just Frankincense too...You can also put the resin into a pitcher of water overnight, then drink that water the next day-Frankincense water-it tastes good!(you can put stevia & lemon juice in it too)

Vega One All in One Nutritional powder Chocolate flavour is high in Titanium(from the hemp seeds)-it also contains many excellent Minus items(detoxifying items)...If you want to take a multivitamin every day that won't interfere with your anticancer protocol, this powder is the one...Get a giant tub & have some when you run out of food & are too tired from hunger to go shopping! (Their sugar free energizer powder with ginger & turmeric is a great booster for when you are first diagnosed & feel run down due to unhappiness-also it lowers Lead levels in the bones)…

BuyWeedOnline.ca sells CBD oil online to Canadians, & you can pay using online banking e-transfer, & the CBD oil will be discreetly & quickly shipped to you for your medical needs…The seller calls himself Ronald, & is trustworthy…It costs about $50 Cdn currency a gram, & is the finest quality, from where it is grown & made & sold legally, in British Columbia, Canada…You take a nail's head amount, & dip it into slightly microwaved peanut butter(a tablespoon), & stir them together, & eat it…If you do not have high cholesterol at all, it will not benefit you greatly…People with low cholesterol, do not really need their cholesterol lowered much further, which is what CBD oil(Cannabidiol) does…This stock is High CBD low THC, for people who do not want to get stoned, but do have Cancer…

Potassium:Stevia, Hawthorne, Coconut water, Bananas, (artificial sweeteners are one molecule sugar with 4 molecules potassium by the way- yes, even the ones that get vilified by natural blogs- biggest danger is overly lowering blood pressure- beta blockers are also potassium- blood pressure lowering drugs)…(Basal cells feed on B12/Taurine/Cobalt-all high blood pressure markers, which Potassium lowers)…Diet sodas have tons of potassium in them by the way…

Potassium: Stevia lowers "Aurum"(from the Grove Body Part Chart), which in layperson's terms is B12, Cobalt, the thing that raises blood pressure, Taurine, but also the thing that bugs are attracted to…Well, in particular, in dogs, they'd call that "heart worm"…The triple negative group would also have high Aurum (B12 blood pressure) levels…As well as several other types of cancers, including those found in people who eat a lot of fish, especially raw fish…Anyways…You can buy giant bags of Stevia & sprinkle it in your food, your drink & even in your dog's food…Not too much-potassium can lower blood pressure so much your heart can stop…If you take too much, or your dog does, then add back some fish to your or his/her diet…

Novel drug:**PNC 27** is made of fruit fly & moth…The fruit fly is biochemically similar to anthocyanin…The moth is similar to saponins…Anthocyanins are like Oxygens, like what you find in things that clean the liver-Milk thistle, dandelion, apricot kernels, goji berries, berries, sundried tomatoes, fresh air…Saponins are like Titaniums-found in Vanilla Beans, Comfrey, Frankincense, chamomile, thyme…Saponins clean out the Lungs & lymph nodes & lower cholesterol…So PNC 27 might be especially effective for people with Liver problems & high cholesterol…

Carbon:Olive oil, Flaxseed oil(the flaxseed in this oil is a Manganese by the way), Grapeseed oil, Baking Soda, any cooking oils

Selenium:Garlic, Garlic pills, Cayenne Pepper, Pancreatic enzymes, Spicy things like Sriracha sauce, lysine, antibiotics, insulin, pepper, MSM (Methylsulfonylmethane) cream(mix MSM with Iodine & apply topically- absorbs better)(Squamous cells eat sugar which Seleniums lower)...

Oxygen:Apricot kernels(grind & put in unsweetened applesauce), Butcher's broom, Arsenicum Album, seeds of apples or lemons or oranges, Blue Flag iris powder or tincture, Fresh air, Apple seeds, Ozone injections, hydrogen peroxide(you can nebulize this too), Eucalyptus oil(nebulize or apply topically)
Apricot kernels oxygenate the Liver & in the brain the Cerebellum...This is very useful in dehydrating tumours, clearing up areas of hypoxia, & also starving microbes that feed on Hydrogen...

Iodine:Iodoral pills 12.5 mg a day, Madagascar periwinkle herb, Vinpocetine pills, Poke root, Kelp tincture, seaweed salad, Japanese food in general, sea vegetables like Arame, Detoxadine(iodine), Tamoxifen, Pau d'arco herb

Copper:Green tea, Copper pills, Licorice root tincture(St. Francis), Gingko Biloba(powerful heavy metal chelator), Chromium, Caffeine(yes, caffeine has Copper in it-GOOD-don't do it if you don't want to but don't argue with me about it, there Is a reason why Starbucks is so successful right now!), Yerba mate, matcha, wheatgrass, ecogallincatechingallate ecgc...Cilantro is a fabulous Copper that is just great to eat!!!! Cilantro extract, liquid chlorophyll, Copper in multivitamins...

"I took various forms of Licorice root for over a year...When I found out that Phosphorus distinguished malignant from benign, I set out to obliterate Phosphorus...I knew Coppers could do that from my studies in Parkinson's disease(which is just excess Phosphorus in the Spleen & Globus Palladus)...My brother helped me choose Licorice root as the Copper I'd use...I had been editing photos to show chemistry of the lump, & could actually see the Phosphorus(looks like tiny purple ants)...I got some St. Francis Licorice root tincture & gulped maybe 1/4 of the bottle...The next day, I took & edited more pictures, & sure enough the purple ants were clearing up...That was when I began to lose my fear & feel like I could win...Later I found some clinical studies that said Licorice root could cause phenotypic reversion- revert malignant back to benign...So my own theories were supported by others...You can live with a giant benign lump indefinitely...Most people set the goal to shrink it, which can be very difficult...But if you set the goal to change its chemistry to benign…Well…" Sari Grove

Gingko Biloba:You can empty a Gingko Biloba capsules onto your pet's wet or dry food to get some Copper into their daily diet…It is a stimulant, so be aware of that…

Cocaine:Cocaine is also a Copper…If you have parasites that have gone up your nose or into your brain from up your nose(aspirating them), then possibly you could snort Cocaine, though it is usually illegal, very expensive, quality is questionable, & can be dangerous…Plastic surgeons use medical grade cocaine when they do nose jobs or nose repair, so you could ask one of them for some for your nasal or brain cancer…

Magnesium:Epsom Salt baths, oral epsom salts(get from your pharmacist), Magnesium pills, Lavender, Glutathione is what they call it sometimes, Whey Protein they call it also, exercise

Fluorine:Parsley, toothpaste(sorry, I was a non-fluoride girl too, believe me…But Fluorine actually unclogs things…In the good old days fluoride was a bit of a miracle…)most large bodies of water have natural fluorine in them go for a swim…Listerine mouth wash, Hydrochloric acid(therapy-drops in water, drink or nebulize)(Melanoma likes to eat the Bismuth family which is lowered by Fluorine including the chemo drug Fluorouracil which can be used topically on melanomas…DIYselfers can find fluorine in many other places, to apply topically & also ingest orally…This is not the time to be anti- fluoride if you have melanomas)…Moringa Oleifera is also a great new Fluorine!

Boron:I have not found a better way to get Boron than in a supplement sorry…I will add something when I find something…The supplement I took had potassium, apple cider vinegar(it's a Zinc), & Boron all at once…Borax is another way to get Boron…You can put 1/4 cup of laundry Borax into your bathwater to get your Boron…For your pet, crush an all Boron supplement pill under a spoon, & stir into their wet or dry food…

Ecstasy(MDMA) is a heroin copycat in a pill that is so strong it acts like Boron…Side effects include profuse sweating for extended periods of time, dry mouth for extended periods of time(like a week or more), trance like state, very very submissive behaviour, paralysis long term(you do not do anything with your life at all), & slavery(you are so submissive you end up caged mentally, or working in an adult entertainment club as a sexual slave, or as a drug addicted user with no funds since you drained them all to pay for your habit)…However, Ecstasy, the street drug in pill form, has applications for prostate & ovarian cancers…It lowers Molybdenum levels in the Cerebral Aqueduct in the brain, & in the Prostate in the male, & in Skene's Gland in the female(the female prostate is called Skene's gland)…It should be used as a last resort…Start with a legal Boron supplement available at Health food stores(Qi Natural Foods at Eglinton & Allen road is an excellent source)…

For everybody: Humaworm is an all around antiparasitic blend…Everyone with any type of Cancer should take it…Here is the link to what is in it https://humaworm.com/formula.html

Ok so there is a short list of ideas…Feel free to substitute…(the following are just some more ideas & examples to consider…)

For example…(these 4 things are in Zenith Herbals Bloodroot capsules)…

Galangal is in the Ginger family=it's a ZINC

Chaparall is in the Selenium family

Graviola is in the Potassium family

Bloodroot-a Manganese

"A Beta Blocker drug is essentially Potassium…It lowers blood pressure…It makes the heart slightly larger, probably due to its anti diuretic effect, so by holding on water the heart swells a bit which lowers overall pressure…Potassiums are actually very useful anticancer tools, in particular for basal cell types,which comprise 75% of the more aggressive types…Graviola for instance is a Potassium…Too much potassium can lower blood pressure excessively & can cause you to be very sluggish…Piece of trivia: artificial sweeteners are 1 molecule sugar & 4 molecules potassium…Stevia is also high in potassium, as is Hawthorn…"(Sari Grove)

The bloodroot capsules work specifically like this: Bloodroot (a Manganese) lowers Iron in the Thymus which makes blood- Iron is a component of both benign & malignant tumours…Galangal(Ginger family) is a Zinc that lowers Lead in the Thyroid gland which builds bone…Chaparral is a Selenium family that lowers blood sugar in the Pancreas…Graviola is a Potassium that lowers Aurum(blood pressure) in the Heart…The Zenith Herbals bloodroot capsules are double strength…So, yes, I think they would be a very helpful component to a serious anticancer regime…

Now that's not all…

The best diet you can choose for an anticancer protocol is a Raw Vegetable diet…

Here's a link to how to do that… **It's a book by a nurse who cured her breast cancer JUST by going raw…Buy it…It is a digital download…Going raw is a big step…Read this book…It got me to go raw…Until I went raw, the herbs were not really working to their full potential…I also lost 50 lbs…50 lbs…Without dieting…(no calorie control, no portion control, not trying to lose weight actually)…(The book is called My Raw food cure & diet secrets by Helen Hecker RN)…**

Ok, next big thing is exercise…Here is something that is free & pretty easy to do…Walk…I started a year & half ago…Just walking…I'd listen to music…I found a nice trail in the city that made me happy…The first time I did the walk it took me something like 3 hours…I was out of shape…Now it takes me maybe an hour & a half…But my distance is almost 12 kilometres now on trail…(trails are harder than sidewalk)…I used to walk maybe 8 kilometres with plenty of breaks to pat people's dogs, chat, take pictures, or maybe stop for a drink or lunch or sit around reading Facebook messsages in the sun…

Walking every day is like a full time job…You will need cute outfits, good running shoes, earphones & a music playing device is helpful if you need motivation(I use the app called Rock My Run-it has playlists of upbeat music pre-chosen so I don't have to choose & I don't get bored…I pay about $5 a month now for their premium service…But I did use it for free for a long time before that…

Walk…Seriously…It is going to take probably 2 hours, maybe longer for a good walk…You will be exhausted at the end…You may not be able to feel your feet-they can feel a little numb at the end of a good walk when you are still out of shape…

Walk…You don't have to walk fast…At all…But do it every single day if you can…I cannot decide which is more important, the diet or the walking…I am guessing maybe the walking…because it fixes depression, anxiety, panic, fear & you get to talk to God who is going to be your very best closest friend while you do all of this…

You don't have to walk with other people & make it a group thing…It is very Zen to walk alone…I smile & say hello to people as I walk by them…They smile back & say

hello…That is pretty good…For socializing…You don't need too much more…(I do try to pat people's dogs though because that really makes me feel happy inside…Don't pat people's dogs without asking permission first…In case the dog is a biter…Doesn't happen often…)

Walk…

You will start to look like an athlete…Your body will get sexy again…People will tell you that you are glowing…

Walk…Walk far…

Ok, that is it for advice now…If you need extra help besides what is on this website or what is in my books(free very small size downloads at NoiseTrade of all our books…(or look for the Free Books page in the Menu of this website for more choices of how to read our books)…oh, I forgot to give you an email address…here it is grove@sent.com…If you need help ask…I got time…

Big Cool Important thing to learn how to do:If you have a lump somewhere & want to see what it looks like at home, whenever you want to, read this post…(I took pictures of my "lump" & edited them myself with this technique & kept track of size & chemistry changes all the way along up to the present…)

Things to consider:

Birth control drugs are made of Calcium & Phosphorus…The vast majority of malignant tumours are made of Calcium & Phosphorus…

Treat all cancers at their most base level as if they are made of Calcium & Phosphorus…That means you need Iodine & Copper for sure…Then find out what body part your tumour is living in…Clean out THAT body part in particular…Use our Chart, The Grove Body Part Chart to decide what to use…For example, if the tumour is in your Liver, see that Oxygen is the Minus, & Hydrogen is the Plus…So you need Oxygen, the Minus to detox the Liver…Choose an Oxygen…Apricot kernels are a great Oxygen for the Liver…

You are what you eat & so is your tumour…If you eat eggs everyday then your tumour will be high in cholesterol(which we call Aluminum on our Chart)…If you eat bread everyday then your tumour will be high in glutens which we call Nitrogen on our Chart…Triple Negative breast cancers tend to be high in those two things…Choline & Glutamate, otherwise known as cholesterol & gluten, otherwise known on the Grove Body Part Chart as Aluminum & Nitrogen…So you need to specifically add the correct Minus element to your protocol…Titanium & Carbon are the Minus elements for that…(but do not neglect the standard procedure for all cancers, Iodine & Copper)…

Iron is a component of both benign & malignant tumours that makes them hard…

Melatonin is in the Bismuth** family & makes a tumour feel bumpy…Bumpy when you feel your lump is NOT good…SMOOTH is what you want our lump to feel like…Though I love melatonin, be very careful how & when & how much you use to help you sleep…Sometimes you just have to sleep…But know that it will make your lump feel bumpy & rough & that scares doctors into saying things like:"You MUST have surgery"…

**(things with fluoride in them remove Bismuth(which makes your lump feel smooth again after you took all that melatonin cause the sleeping was so delicious)…Dentists have liquid swish drinks with fluoride in them…Just saying…)

In response to a question about Caffeine…

"Caffeine is just another source of Copper…It is chemically opposite to Phosphorus…Birth control drugs are Calcium & Phosphorus which cause a heavy load on the Adrenal Gland & the Spleen…That heavy load is why people are walking around with compromised immune systems right now…(there are other reasons of course too, but the birth control drug pressure on our bodies is possibly the most significant new factor since the 60s…) Acquired Immune Deficiency Syndrome (AIDS) is just adrenal gland failure…Which is why the Iodine family is crucial- it cleans out the Calcium from the Adrenal gland…But yes, too much of anything, either way, can cause imbalance…Which is why you have to be careful not to overdo a detox program, why you should cheat a little on everything people say, take detox vacations where you slack off, & why you may have to take some " opposite" stuff later to fix the fact that you were overzealous…Too much caffeine or Copper family & you may need to start drinking Kefir to put back some of the good Phosphorus you got rid of…Coffee enemas are a way to get Copper-I didn't use them myself because I was on a raw plant based diet with tons of oil & apple cider vinegar & my colon was pretty darn cleaned out just from that…Also I am lazy… But some people feel they are integral…(Gee, now I think I should try them…hmm…) If you are uncomfortable with something, it's not right for you…Use your spidey senses…A billion people will tell you to quit caffeine…New studies show coffee & tea are great at fighting cancers…

(this person asking had already had some surgery done)-But again, for you, after surgery, it may be too harsh…Surgery means you need to do a lot of repairing too…A nice thing to do which repairs is to drink Aloe Vera juice every day…It heals up where they have cut, but also does some cleaning out work…Mix it with Mangosteen juice or Acai juice for some flavour…"

Ovarian Cysts; Buy Dr. Reckeweg, R38, & R39…Each bottle costs about $25 dollars…Take a generous swig of each…If you are lucky, the cysts will fall out in the toilet when you pee 48 hours later…Repeat every few months to make sure all are gone…I would also do several rounds in the case of Ovarian cancer since cancer develops from cysts…(the Dr. Reckeweg formulas for ovarian cysts contain bees! Very high dose Manganese which causes Iron to lower & cysts detach!)

If you have a brain tumour or brain cancer, see the Grove Brain Body Part Chart…Find the closest brain part to where your tumour is, then find the corresponding Minus element to take for that part…(see top of page for newer brain part chart)

Brain Parts	Body Parts	Minus	Plus
Minus	" There are two	female ♀	Male ♂
Plus	sides to every	-	+
12 Brain Part Locations	body part "...	chromosome	chromosome
Frontal Lobe -right / Frontal Lobe left +	Thyroid left Thyroid right	Zinc-1	Lead+12
Motor Cortex- right / Motor Cortex+left	Thymus left Thymus right	manganese-2	Iron+11
Parietal Lobe - right / Parietal Lobe+left	leftLung & Lymph Node / Lung & Lymph Node right	Titanium-3	Aluminum+10
Medulla Oblongata -Top / Medulla Oblongata+bottom	Heart left Heart right	Potassium-4	Aurum+9
Pons -Top / Pons + Bottom	Kidney left Kidney right	Carbon-5	Nitrogen+8
Occipital Lobe- / Occipital Lobe+left	Pancreas left Pancreas right	Selenium-6	Sugar +7
Cerebellum - Right / Cerebellum+left	Liver bottom Liver top	Oxygen-7	Hydrogen+6
Pituitary Gland- Right / Pituitary Gland+left	Adrenal Gland bottom / topAdrenal Gland	Iodine-8	Calcium+5
Globus Palladus-front / Hypothalamus+back	bottom Spleen Spleen top	Copper-9	Phosphorus+4
Broca's Area - front / Wernicke's Area+Back	Gallbladder bottom top Gallbladder	Magnesium-10	Mercury+3
Temporal Lobe- Right / Pineal Gland+left	Colon bottom Colon top	Fluorine-11	Bismuth+2
Corpus Callosum -front / Cerebral Aqueduct+back	Skene's Gland ♂ / ♀ Prostate Gland	Boron-12	Molybdenum+1

copyright GroveCanada2015

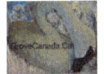

Grove Brain & Body Part Chart

Anti-parasitics:Unda 17 is a Swedish liquid mix that helps to get rid of parasites…

Artemesia Complex by Knowledge Products helps to get rid of old dead parasite shells after you have done several rounds of a regular antiparasitic protocol(wormwood, black walnut hull, clove- is the 3 part protocol Dr. Hulda Clark invented for that)…Some people use diatomaceous earth to get rid of parasites-I did not try this but many say it is great)…

Parasites & Cancer & Candida seem to all go hand in hand & are perhaps interchangeable…My theory is the Salmonella Typhi Bacterium(Typhus) is to blame…I write about that in one of my books…(Book 3)…

lymph detox deodorant recipe: 1 tablespoon organic corn starch, 1 tablespoon baking soda, 2-3 tablespoons organic vegetable glycerin-ok this is the salve base…To this add your favourite essential oils, frankincense, pink grapefruit, orange, lemon, clove, coriander, thyme, eucalyptus, mint…Apply to underarms daily…Rub on parts of the body that need detox attention, like varicose veins, lumpy areas, sore areas…

E-Cadherin is A Titanium marker…Titaniums break down Aluminum/cholesterol…Statin drugs are Titanium…In metaplastic breast cancer, e-cadherin an inhibitor of change in cancer, may be low…Which is why the Titanium Statin family is useful there…Also lowering Aluminum cholesterol levels in other ways…Hulled hemp seeds are a nice natural Statin…

Epidermal growth factor receptor (egfr) is an Aluminum/ cholesterol that is opposite to e-Cadherin in nature…

Estrogen markers are Phosphorus…they need Copper…

Progesterone markers are Calcium…They need Iodines…

Her2 markers are Hydrogen…They need Oxygens like apricot kernels…

Additional Notes:

"Titanium is found in all statin drugs, Mint leafs, baby aspirin, CBD oil, Frankincense essential oil/Boswellia serrata supplements, comfrey, chamomile…No not the heavy metal!!! In tumour markers Titanium is called E-Cadherin…If levels are low that is very Not good…Aggressive cancers have low e-cadherin…So yup, take something in that family…Also lower cholesterol/Aluminum intake(not the heavy metal again)…Eggs are cholesterol…(if you are taking any calcium supplements at all)Yes stop the calcium…Stop the calcium…stop the calcium…All tumours whether benign or malignant have calcium…Birth control drugs are calcium(& phosphorus btw)…Progesterone means calcium…" love sari

Titanium is also in Iscador(injections)

Sari Grove
Boswellia capsules, Iodoral pills, Licorice root tincture, Bloodroot capsules(Zenith herbals), raw plant based diet, no sugar, no dairy, no gluten, walk 2 hrs daily, Boron. Apple cider vinegar, ginkgo biloba, Vinpocetine, Mugwort, green tea, apricot kernels, Hepa plus by Usana, Paragone antiparasitics, hawthorn, frankincense (chew the nuggets then spit out the gym), vitamin d3 , vitamin c, ginger root simmer into tea…

p.s.On my chart, substitute the word Sulphur(if you still see it) for the word Sugar…It's a mistake…I am human…It's a big one though, please forgive me…

How to get rid of a breast cancer lump tutorial on Tildee by Sari Grove…

Risky business: Breast implants(3x more likely to die of lung cancer, 2x more likely to die of brain cancer, immune system malfunction, chronic fatigue, infection, mold, rare lymphoma…), Any birth control drug(try Vitus Agnus Castus instead- herbal celibacy inducer), Acrylic nails & acrylic nail salons (BPA is highly phosphorus estrogenic)…

***Generally you take Artemisia, also called Wormwood, while also taking Black walnut hull tincture, & Clove capsules…This is the 3 part antiparasitic protocol designed by Dr. Hulda Clark, & they are very effective all together…The parasite theory of Cancer is very pervasive & I believe everybody should participate in the 3 part strategy…

Can I black salve my Lymph node tumour under my armpit?

The reason there is reticence here is because the lymph nodes under the armpit are such a sensitive area pain wise…So philosophically, many would try all the other possible lymph detox methods first, Moxibustion, acupuncture, lymph detox massage, raw diet, essential oils topically & orally, daily very long walks for exercise to get everything going- just everything you can possibly think of, saunas, steam baths, nebulizing eucalyptus oil, baking soda therapy, Hydrochloric acid therapy, mega dosing vitamin c- you want to throw the kitchen sink at it, before deciding to black salve there- because it is such a tender area…

Note: Black salve refers to Bloodroot salve, A Manganese thing…

Black salve capsules (Zenith Herbals) contain double strength bloodroot/ manganese, galangal/zinc, chaparral/selenium, graviola/potassium…A great way to get someone going in their alternative anticancer treatment in just one pill a day!(you can take more)…

CBD oil(I got mine from buyweedonline.ca): "What I was saying, is that if you are already very low cholesterol, it doesn't change things as significantly as someone who is high cholesterol…THC acts like a cholesterol lowering drug, which aggressive tumours feed on…For someone like me, I was able to get effect from eating hulled hemp seeds daily, hemp oil, Frankincense oil & chewing Frankincense tears(you spit the gum out after)…You can even chew vanilla beans which has a similar effect…Aspirin acts in the same way too…"

Alternatives to CBD oil (Titanium group): Hulled hemp seeds from Whole Foods or pretty much anywhere, Hemp oil too- any health food store…Frankincense essential oil is always around- topical quality…Plenty of people in these groups(Facebook groups), say for internal Frankincense oil , to order from so & so brand because it is purer & they are probably right…Frankincense tears can be found locally though I dont know where you live- you can also find a plethora of suppliers for the Frankincense tears online…Just get the nice fresh yellow looking ones if you are going to chew them…Vanilla beans often come in a small clear tube at your grocery store…You can scrape out the brown goop from the bean after cutting them open in two, & just eat that, then chew the pod until there is no more flavour & spit that out…(you can swallow the pods too- perfectly edible)…

Just the basics:

You need an Iodine in your mix, some Licorice root tincture to prevent & reverse spread, & a Manganese…(You can get herb forms of these three things from Herbies Herbs in Toronto- they will ship to you for cheap…You can order Madagascar Periwinkle herb(Iodine), Licorice root herb(Copper), & Mugwort herb(Manganese)…Order like the small amounts to start…Take 1/3 of a cup of each herb, dump all in a pot, cover with water & more, simmer 15 minutes, & drink the black liquid…This was my DIY chemo recipe…It is very good…(not tastewise sorry)…But it covers the basic bases…Not an expensive protocol…Easy to do…

Frontal lobe...Thyroid
Motor Cortex...Thymus
Parietal Lobe...Lungs & Lymph Nodes

Medulla Oblongata...Heart

Pons...Kidneys

Occipital Lobe...Pancreas

Cerebellum...Liver

Pituitary Gland...Adrenal Gland

Globus Palladus/Hypothalamus Spleen

Broca's/Wernicke's Area...Gallbladder

Temporal Lobe/Pineal gland...Colon

Corpus Callossum/Cerebral
Aqueduct...Prostate/Skene's Gland
www.GroveCanada.Ca

Grove Brain Part Chart

Comments about THC, CBD oil, Cannabis, Marijuana & various forms of cancer...

THC lowers cholesterol which aggressive cancers like to feed on...

A triple positive person may respond to THC, but may not have the significant results because their cancer is not feeding on their cholesterol, which may in fact be low already...

I believe that THC is beneficial across the board, just more beneficial to those with higher cholesterol levels...

For those who say their tumours grew while on THC, I think it was not that the THC fed the cancer, just that it eradicated something that was not a problem to begin with…So the cancer just continued to feed on the hormones it was already feeding on…

Many people while doing a THC substance as medicine do several other things that influence outcome-they do it exclusively as a wonder cure, they stop exercising, they eat because it makes them hungrier, they sleep all day…Then when they check their tumour they say it has grown & blame the THC…I do not think this is a fair or correct evaluation of the process…

p.s. Since THC also constipates, this affects their evaluation of outcome…

Sari Grove
EGFR Epidermal growth factor receptor is the Cancer marker that the THC products target…Very effectively…EGFR is a cholesterol type marker…Often over expressed in lung cancer but also in aggressive breast cancers(like the triple negatives)…

While you are sourcing your oil, you should be doing all the things in that same family of medicine…For example, eating a giant bowl of hulled hemp seeds for breakfast…Chewing & swallowing the spice called Clove…Chewing & swallowing the Vanilla Bean(they come in tubes at grocery stores)…Ingesting Frankincense oil…You can chew Frankincense tears(the nuggets) too- but spit out the gum when the flavour is gone(minty)…Over the counter hemp oil shots(mix with apple cider vinegar for taste)…All these things lower the EGFR market-epidermal growth factor receptor…In another category of medicine to stop spread & reverse it: hit wheatgrass, spirulina, liquid chlorophyll, green tea extract & tea, matcha, Licorice root extract, chromium, boron, Yerba mate…This family stops spread…

The missing pieces:

(again!)

Have you been doing any of the following category? :wheatgrass, spirulina, liquid chlorophyll, matcha, green tea extract, green tea, chromium, boron, yerba mate, plant caffeines, licorice root extract? (Note: The studies about Copper are actually about Ceruloplasmin which is a Copper binder- its opposite, Phosphorus- so if you are restraining on the Copper family because of that flawed study, know that it is wrong & you absolutely need Copper to stop & reverse spreading…This might be your missing piece because it seems many were misled by that one misreported badly written study…

1)On the first page of this website is a post that explains how to see under your skin with your own camera & a simple free editing program… If you have cancer anywhere in your body, or you are worried & want to prevent getting cancer, or you have had surgery & want to see what is happening-please go to that post & watch the short video & learn how to take & edit your own pictures…

For places like the lungs, you can take pictures from the front or from the back(you may need help from a friend for your back-though with a bathroom mirror & some stretching I have done it)…Make sure your picture is very close-up, in good light, & hold still for a few seconds before pressing the take picture button…

*****If you only have an iPhone** do not despair…Go to the App store…Download the **Puffin app**…That allows you to access the Fotoflexer(it uses Flash) program on an iPhone…If you use the **Camera+** app for iPhone to take your picture, the picture will be better(more clarity, & you can edit it to make it sharper before you upload to Fotoflexer online)…**Photoshop Express** is another editing app for iPhone that I use to make pictures even more sharp before uploading to Fotoflexer…

Take a picture before & the day after taking a new alternative treatment…That will tell you if it is working or not…Be aware that stress & exercise initially causes a lump to swell up soon after exercising, but then the next day it will be much much smaller…So wait to take your pictures after exercising or stress…(this is why diagnostic pictures are often so disappointing-the stress & exercise of getting to the appointment causes lumps to swell temporarily…)

(Warning:The path that I took was to avoid all surgery…No chemo, no radiation, no Tamoxifen…So the following post is from that perspective, that bias…

This path is NOT(**I may have been a little harsh here-you can use this program-just be more gentle with yourself**) for people who have done surgery, chemo, radiation or tamoxifen…You can still learn from reading, but this path is too severe for those who have already gone through the severity of conventional medicine…

It is VERY difficult to do a detox after surgery because after surgery your body needs to heal, to feel loved & to be fed…Chemo can be very debilitating…Radiation can be something to get used to-not in a good way…So once again, the following is for people who are trying to avoid cut, poison, burn as they call it…If you have any of the cut, poison, burn options, then you need to go slower…gentler…easier…Ok?)

About that:" Yes…I put that warning in because once people have had surgery or radiation or chemo, they've already covered some of their bases already…

Radiation will have covered what I call the "Zinc" category- so that is the whole Vitamin D3, megadose Vitamin C, ginger root, galangal – all that stuff that lowers Lead levels in bone & Thyroid gland…

Chemo is usually in the Iodine category- so you will have already have gotten a fair dose of that if your chemo was pretty standard…So you may have already covered two bases…If you have had any surgeries or biopsies, you may have some repair & healing to do…

Which means be careful with the whole blood thinning Titanium category like CBD oil, Iscador, Frankincense, aspirin- that category can increase bleediness & prevent healing of wounds, so that has to be taken into account…

Comment about being careful about what you read on the Internet:

Yeah!Like with Cloves…What they say about things being estrogenic is just plain wrong…On the internet, you get one bad study poorly written & the whole planet just copies the info…Licorice root does not boost estrogen, neither does Red Clover, Gingko

Biloba, Dong Quai, Black Cohosh- yet you will find all sorts of wrong about them…Coppers kill cancer, but one dumb study misreported the word Ceruloplasmin as Copper, so everybody copied & now the internet says Copper is bad…They are referring to Ceruloplasmin as Copper, but it is not…It is a Copper BINDER…That means its opposite…The mistake is rampant, & can kill people…The one night shift study in melatonin & cancer is so poorly set up & flawed, yet the whole internet is ablaze with untruths about melatonin being anticancer…The chemistry just doesn't work…Fluorine is used often in chemo for colon, lung, breast cancer- a drug called Fluorouracil, but fluorine gets a bad rap every day…People forget that all these so called clinical trials can get easily published on medical sites with just a credit card payment…

Melatonin & Progesterone:

Sari Grove

Melatonin raises serotonin…Serotonin raises estrogen…But Dr. Veronique Desaulniers recommends it in her book & there is a study of night shift workers that people cite…The flaw there is: Dr. V. used black salve to remove her tumour…It contains the caustic Zinc Chloride which would lower melatonin levels exponentially & raise fluorine levels…That would have made melatonin very attractive to her biochemically…It worked for her, & now it's in her program…But not everybody has done black salve…So their levels will be very very different…Same with the night shift worker study…Night shift workers would have radically high fluorine & radically low melatonin…So it worked for them too…But not everyone is a night shift worker…Those are serious biases…As long as you know why you are doing something, then that is safe…But thinking something like melatonin is anticancer based on the night shift worker study or the experience of someone who used black salve(no offence intended), is naive…Personally I love melatonin…Great sleep…But I don't think it is anticancer…I do think sleep is important…Melatonin made my lump gritty & bumpy…When I quit it became smooth & more even…It was definitely not anticancer for me…But I will take it when I am insomniac …I know how to antidote its effect too if I have to…Progesterone acts like Calcium in the body…You could drink milk & get a similar effect for less money…Or bathe in it(milk bath)…Will make lump grow(but not malignant- just size)…

In response to a question about Hodgkins Lymphoma:(People friend me on Facebook then we can chat via Facebooks messaging service-here is an excerpt…)

- You should do a 30 day run of Humaworm…It is an antiparasitic remedy that is probably the best on the market… For hodgkins lymphoma you need to specifically address the Liver…So-Apricot kernels(an Oxygen that lowers Hydrogen in the Liver), Milk thistle, Dandelion greens, Goji berries, all berries, sundried tomatoes-if you want a supplement there is Hepa Plus by Usana which is very good…Burdock root is excellent…I see you already take milk thistle…Great…Take more! (Empty supplements out of their capsules & put them in a glass & add some liquid & drink-they will hit you faster & better than inside the capsules-plus there is less swallowing to do that way)…I dont see any Coppers in your list…(sorry, this laptop is acting up-there may be typos-it wants to type in a different language-will try to fix this soon)…For Coppers, I love Licorice root-extract, capsules, herb, tea-get alot…It kills malignancy, stops spread & reverses damage…Also wheatgrass, spirulina, liquid chlorophyll, chlorella, cilantro, fennel, green tea, black tea, coffee, st. johns wort…http://grovecanada.ca/so-you-want-to-go-alternative-with-your-cancer-treatment-but-you-dont-know-where-to-start/

So you want to go "alternative" with your cancer treatment but you don't know where to start… I…

So you want to go "alternative" with your cancer treatment but you don't know where to start... I can help with that... I will try & make this as

grovecanada.ca

- 17:34

Sari Grove

Id like you to take some pictures, close up, & edit them yourself using my instructions in this blog post…Do the Fotoflexer edit…Then go to the instructions for malignancy to the Lunapic blogpost…Then you will be able to see what is happening chemically now & also how much malignancy or cancer is there…Then we will know better how to proceed…Both are easy & free to do…The second one is longer(15 steps)…The first is only 4 steps…Take pictures where you are worried about…

- 17:34

Sari Grove

http://grovecanada.ca/how-to-see-a-lump-in-your-breast-by-sari-grove/

How to see a lump in your breast(or anywhere else)…by Sari Grove | Artists innovating in the…

Instructions for how to see a lump under your skin in your body: How to do it…(Basic Instructions) Take a picture with your camera set to Macro Flash on

grovecanada.ca

Dangerous items:Anything in the PLUS element column could be dangerous to someone with Cancer…

If you still have Cancer present, for example, Bentonite clay(an Aluminum like Zeolite), which repairs damage, can reactivate malignancy that is relatively dormant…Please wait until you are ALL CLEAR before beginning a repair protocol with bentonite clay…

Dangerous if you still have Malignancy present:HRT:Hormone replacement therapies like the Lifewave patches, Chasteberry Vitex for panic due to excess Copper usage, Wild Yam supplements for wound repair & replacement of sexuality loss(also Aluminum), Soy Isoflavones(a Phosphorus) which can relieve arthritic like damage due to taking too much glutathione/magnesium supplements or exercising too much…

Shaving:Cutting yourself brings Hydrogen in loads to the area of the wound…This can feed Liver flukes, which can stay relatively asymptomatic in your body, but present one day as Shingles rash when you cut or injure yourself somewhere…Chronic fatigue syndrome, Epstein-Barr disease, chicken pox, Herpes, Liver Cancers-are all related to Liver flukes…Treat any of those problems with an Oxygen like Eucalyptus(you can nebulize it), or Burdock root, or very very fresh Oxygenated air walks or mountain climbing or skiing or snowboarding…Or Liquid Milk thistle…You will need to heal the wound as well…However, just because you have healed the wound, does not mean you have killed the Liver fluke…In some ways the rash may be a gift-it tells you flukes are present & you need to go hard & heavy on the Oxygens…Apricot kernels in unsweetened applesauce are a great start…(The Humaworm anti-parasitic protocol has also been successful at removing Liver flukes…)

Surgery:Is cutting as well, which brings Hydrogen to the wound area…Hydrogen can feed any stray Cancer cells…Post-operatively, you may want to Oxygenate your diet to clean your Liver out fully…A Liver cleanse kit is a good idea…Or you could do this before surgery, & maybe be able to avoid surgery by killing off parasites Before doing something more invasive…A lump is a response to a wound…often a wound is caused by a parasite eating into your skin…They create a hole…Then your body sends in a repair team which may cause a lump to appear…However, the lump is not necessarily the cancer…The cancer is the creature eating holes in your body…So removing a lump may not remove the cancer…Your first priority should be to kill the parasites…You can live with lumps…

Facebook comments:Licorice root murders the thing they call Cancer, the Phosphorus, the estrogen creature…I am a huge fan…It has few side effects, is cheap, you can take a lot, & it is easy to get in many formats- hugely effective…Iodine shrinks Calcium which is the bulk of lumps, it also corrects many problems that people with Cancer don't talk about like gender dysphoria, weight problems, & lack of sex drive & sexiness…Green tea is an excellent daily drink & plenty should be drunk…Works like the Licorice root…Rosemary is an Oxygen, so it dehydrates tumours which can cause excellent & very fast shrinkage which is very encouraging, it also is good for the Liver…In my work, The Grove Body Part Chart, I sort elements into each body part, tell you where you can find them in the real world, then you choose the ones you prefer…Oxygens are important anticancer…If you happen to live on a Rosemary patch, you might choose that as your preferred Oxygen…I am taking liquid Milk thistle right now as my Oxygen because I can't seem to get apricot kernels anymore locally…Also I am tired of swallowing pills…I love essential oils but my wallet tired of them…So you have many choices…Hepa Plus by Usana is an excellent Liver supplement which contains several good Oxygens…Thunder God vine is another Oxygen…Of course fresh air daily walks might be the best Oxygen…

(brain Tumour at back of head near neck)Diffuse intrinsic pontine glioma…

This brain tumour lives in the Pons…Which controls the Kidneys…So the blockage can be alleviated by removing all glutens from the diet, & increasing Carbons which are all the oils…So Castor oil packs, Flaxseed oil orally, & massages in Grapeseed or Apricot oils to increase total body flow…Frankincense oil crosses the blood brain barrier- so application at back of head near top of neck nightly as well as oral drops…Liquid Iodine…Licorice root extract…Both orally daily…No sugar, no dairy, pull away from meat…

Contradictions:The word phytoestrogen should not be used to describe many of the substances…Flaxseed for instance is a Manganese that lowers Iron in the Thymus that makes blood…Soybeans on the other hand, are a Phosphorus thing, that does actually raise estrogen in the Spleen…Seaweed is an Iodine that lowers Calcium in the Adrenal Gland, & like all Iodines, is closest to Tamoxifen & the other drugs in that category- though technically Calcium is not estrogen but progesterone-so saying even Tamoxifen is anti-estrogenic is not exactly precise…True anti-estrogens are things that lower Phosphorus-which is the most important family the Copper family, which includes- Licorice root, spirulina, chlorella, chlorophyll, cilantro/ coriander, chicory, coffee, tea, green tea, fennel…I think the majority of predisposition to cancers is caused by the Calcium Phosphate based birth control drugs, & then chemical constituents in our environment-which lead to attracting parasites, which then get called the ominous cancer…Greater emphasis needs to be placed on antiparasitics(Humaworm is an excellent 30 day one- for pets too)…

Melatonin:raises blood sugar, raises estradiol-I do not recommend Melatonin at all as part of an anticancer protocol…(despite all the nebulous night shift worker studies & studies of "blind" people, which by the way, blindness can be caused by so many different causes that a study that refers just to blind people should be red flagged immediately…) Also melatonin is chemically opposite to Fluorine which IS used anticancer frequently…THAT alone should tell you that melatonin is Not anticancer…That its opposite is used for Colon, Breast, Lung & other Cancers…

How to see a lump in your breast(or anywhere else)...by Sari Grove

by Sari - Monday, June 22, 2015

http://grovecanada.ca/how-to-see-a-lump-in-your-breast-by-sari-grove/

Before word:There are 2 main Editing techniques mentioned here...One is the Fotoflexer edit that looks at biochemistry...This will tell you what some of your imbalances are, & will help you to focus on what exactly to correct for health...The second is a Lunapic edit that ONLY looks for malignancy...Here is the link to the full instructions for the Lunapic edit...http://grovecanada.ca/checking-only-for-malignancyphosphorus-after-looking-at-a-lump-or-where-a-lump-was-or-just-checking-under-the-skin-somewhere/ Note:If you are eating lots of Phosphorus foods including cottage cheese, Kefir, Yogurt, or cheeses, then you could get a false positive for malignancy in Lunapic...Cease eating all those foods for 3 days & see how your pictures look then...

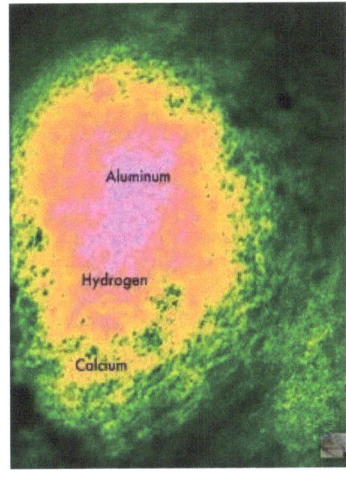

An example of a Fotoflexer edit to see chemistry of a lump...

https://humaworm.com/ordernow.0.html.0.html *Humaworm is an antiparasitic that you take for 30 days...2 capsules morning, 2 capsules evening...If you have Cancer take it...Also give to your pets...And anyone else you have been in contact with...This is not an affiliate link at all...Sari Grove *(please say thank you to Marnie Newton on Facebook for introducing us to Humaworm…Without her research, we would still be having to buy single supplements to make up our recipes…Not to mention, forgetting to add Marshmallow, a demulcent, a Carbon on the Grove Body Part Chart, that softens & helps excrete GMO glutens that can cause physical blockages in the Kidneys, preventing traditional antiparasitics from doing their job)…

Instructions for how to see a lump under your skin in your body:

How to do it…(Basic Instructions)

Take a picture with your camera set to Macro Flash on about 4 inches away(with iPhone camera set to HDR on, iPad cameras & even pretty crummy cameras WILL work!)…

Too close & the flash will be too strong(so get close, then back off so the Flash doesn't ruin the picture-4-5 inches-take a few shots at different distances)…

Camera notes:if you use an iPhone or other Mobile camera, they are set to brighter because most mobile shots are in dark rooms-so your final picture will be brighter-**so you don't necessarily need Flash, & you might not need Macro setting either**…(play with settings to see which pictures give best results…)

Regular Digital Cameras:Do better with **Flash setting On**, & if you can **set the LENS to MACRO** which means it can see detail close-up very well…

*You can Message Sari Grove on Facebook & upload a test picture there & discuss results there with Sari if you want help…(philosophically GroveCanada.ca is a Do It Yourself site, & our books encourage Do It Yourselfing as much as possible…So please do not consider Sari or anyone else to be a replacement for your own expertise…You are the Doctor of your own body, do not give that power away!)

http://grovecanada.ca/so-you-want-to-go-alternative-with-your-cancer-treatment-but-you-dont-know-where-to-start/When you know your results, see this post to understand what things you can do to correct any imbalances you see or malignancies…

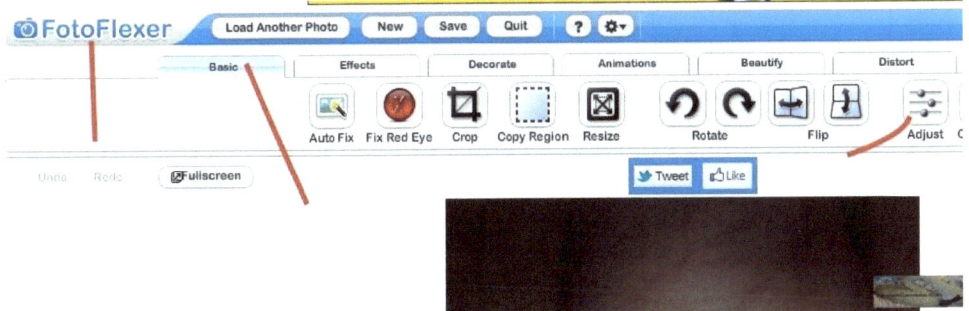

Upload to Fotoflexer.com then in Basic choose Adjust

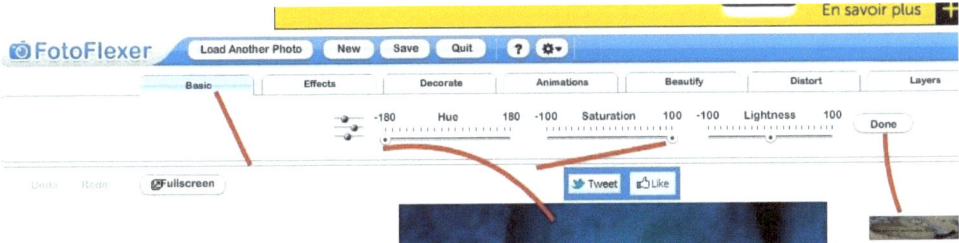

Move HUE all the way to left, Move Saturation all the way to right…

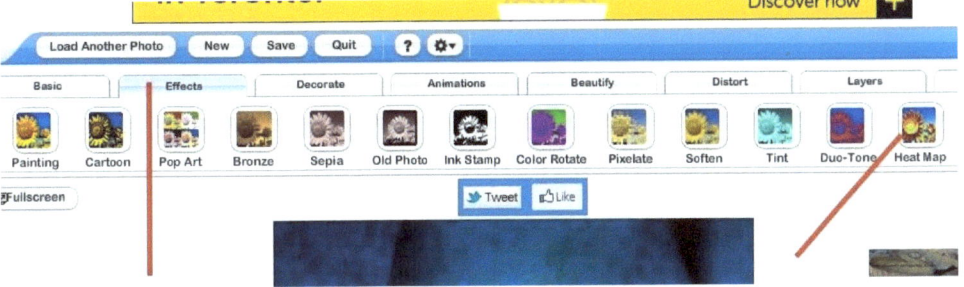

In EFFECTS choose Heat Map(click MORE at top to see Heat map as a choice)

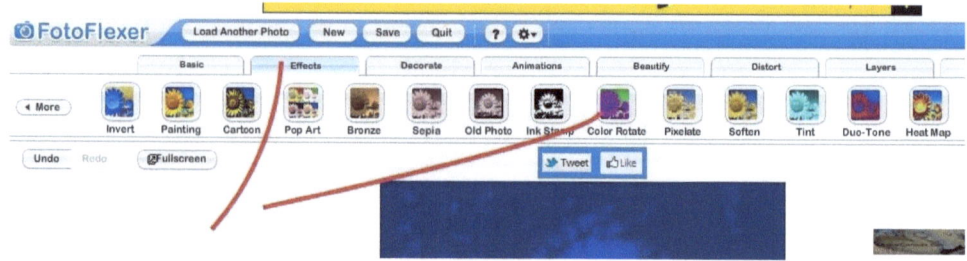

After Applying Heat map, go to COLOR ROTATE, click APPLY as well, then SAVE you are DONE!

4 Easy steps:

1)Upload to http://www.Fotoflexer.com...

2)In Basics adjust Hue(all the way to the left, the slider) & Saturation(move this slider all the way to the right)...

3)In Effects choose Heat Map...

4)Then choose Color Rotate...

(Second editing method)****In Lunapic.com Best Method for checking for Malignancy!

http://www.lunapic.com IF YOU REALLY WANT TO CHECK FOR PHOSPHORUS(malignancy) up close:

Follow these steps...

In Adjust:
click adaptive equalize, apply
click sharpen, slider all the way to right(100%), apply
click color saturation, slider all the way to right, apply
contrast-5x (click this 5 times slowly, wait in between for it to fully load), apply
IN Filters:
thermal effect, apply
HDR lighting, apply

back In Adjust:
adjust light levels—contrast slider to left, highlights slider to left, shadows sliders to left
(all down(to left)), apply
adjust colors:
click the swap red green button
click swap green blue button
click swap blue red button,apply
Normalize, apply,

DONE! (in this edit in Lunapic you are looking for purple Phosphorus only…Any purple is
Phosphorus, malignancy…(Treat with Coppers like licorice root tincture/extract)

Here is the blog post that explains the malignancy edit in Lunapic with a video & more…

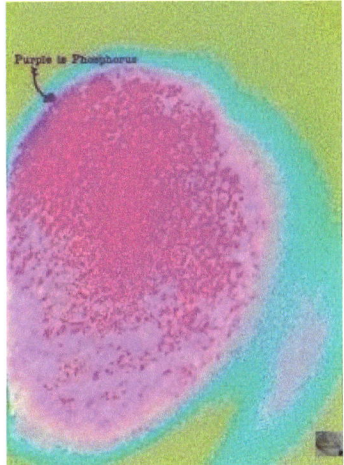

Here is what the look for malignancy edit looks like in
Lunatic, see blog post for more how to…

Ok, back to basics…(The Fotoflexer edit)

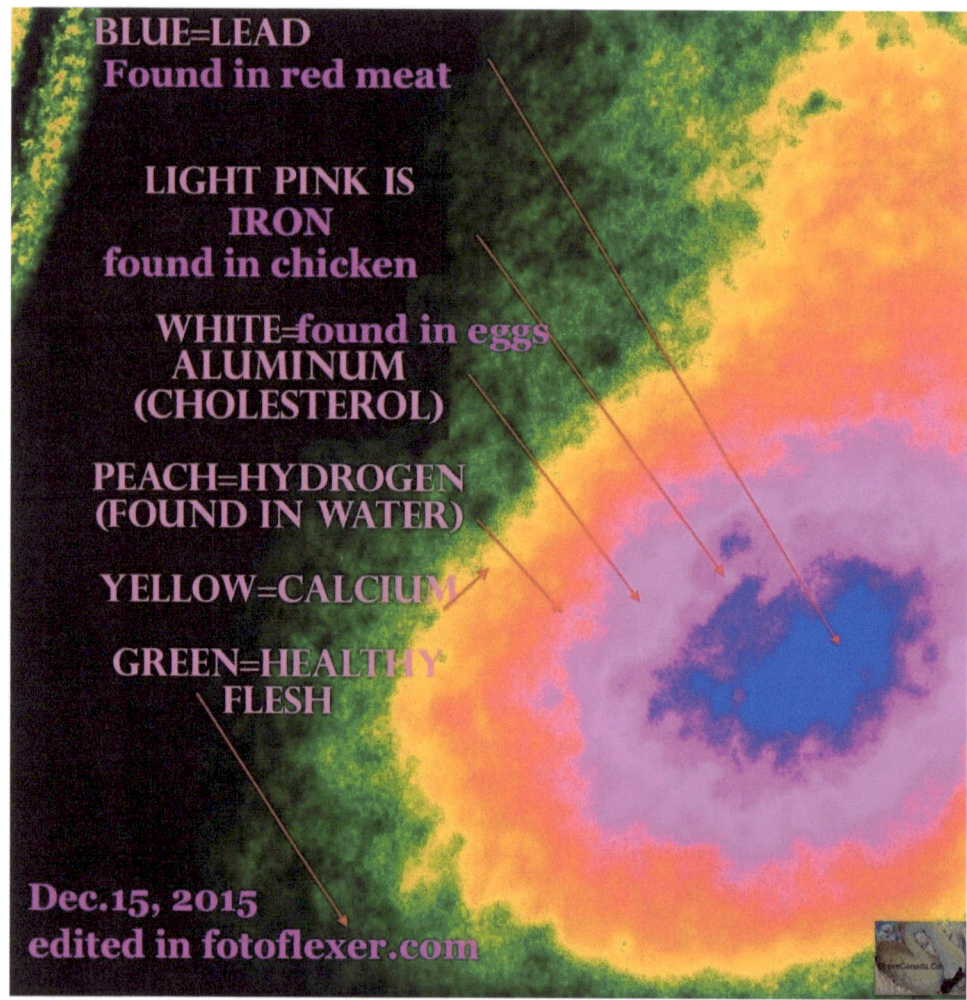

BLUE=LEAD
Found in red meat

LIGHT PINK IS
IRON
found in chicken

WHITE=found in eggs
ALUMINUM
(CHOLESTEROL)

PEACH=HYDROGEN
(FOUND IN WATER)

YELLOW=CALCIUM

GREEN=HEALTHY
FLESH

Dec.15, 2015
edited in fotoflexer.com

What did you see in your edited picture?

Blue is lead(You will get Blue after drinking alcohol the night before or eating red meat)-antagonize with Zinc family like Camu Camu powder for Vitamin C...

Pink(this ring will be right around the Blue Lead) is Iron(you will see Iron after eating chicken) antagonize with a Manganese supplement...

White(it is also slightly pinkish) is Aluminum(Aluminum is cholesterol in the real world)...Antagonize with with Titanium like Boswellia capsules(Frankincense)...
Peach is Hydrogen(you drank ice or water-Necrosis which is characterized by Hypoxia is also excess Hydrogen))...Antagonize with Oxygens like Apricot Kernels...
Dark spots are Phosphorus(You will see Phosphorus after eating cheese, yogurt, Kefir, cottage cheese)(Phosphorus looks like tiny ants)...Antagonize with Licorice root tincture(a Copper)...
Yellow is Calcium...antagonize with Iodine like Iodoral pills 12.5 mg a day...

Green is normal tissue Yay!

Warning:DARK GREEN spots or blobs is Phosphorus...Phosphorus is what makes a lump malignant...You want to clear your lump picture of all those dark green spots...COPPER cleans out Phosphorus...Use the search feature on the website to find out more about how things work, the grove body part chart, our free books, how to download them from Smashwords, & just anything else I might have written about...

http://www.ncbi.nlm.nih.gov/pmc/articles/PMC3702614/ This complicated sounding study basically supports what I have been saying, which is that licorice root is great at getting at breast cancer(& other cancers)...I took licorice tincture first...(later, capsules, the tea, boiled the herb, then just swallowed the herb raw)...Licorice root is a COPPER...(like Ginkgo Biloba, caffeine, green tea, Matcha tea, wheatgrass)...

How the Grove Body Part Chart relates to your lump pictures:The PLUS elements start at LEAD, then IRON, then ALUMINUM, then AURUM, then Nitrogen, Sugar, Hydrogen, Calcium, Phosphorus, Mercury, Bismuth, Molybdenum...

So...When you look at your FOTOFLEXER edited lump picture, the elements will start in the MIDDLE of the LUMP, & work outwards in CONCENTRIC circles...

So Lead(blue in Fotoflexer) should be in the middle, then Pink Iron, then Whitish pink Aluminum, then....Calcium, Phosphorus...NOT all elements can be seen easily in Fotoflexer...

Aurum(B12 which attracts bugs & raises blood pressure), Nitrogen(all glutens & GMO glutens & breads & pastas will block up Kidneys causing physical blockages to getting rid of parasites-Marshmallow helps unblock those blocks since it is a Carbon), Sugar, Mercury & Molybdenum are not easily seen in Fotoflexer...

Phosphorus is also a bit hard to distinguish, which is why we came up with the LUNAPIC editing process which ONLY looks for Phosphorus which indicates malignancy(an alien life form in your body)...Phosphorus can also indicate high consumption of Phosphorus foods, so please cease eating Phosphorus foods for at least 3 days prior to checking your photographs if you don't want to freak out too much at all the Phosphorus purple you will see...If you have been on the Budwig diet(which includes Phosphorus based cottage cheese), you will have to refrain from the cottage cheese for a longer time in order to avoid false positives...

Grove Body Part Chart

Organ	Minus -F Element	Plus +M Element
Thyroid	Zinc -1	Lead +12
Thymus	Manganese -2	Iron +11
Lungs & Lymph Nodes	Titanium -3	Aluminum +10
Heart	Potassium -4	Aurum +9
Kidneys	Carbon -5	Nitrogen +8
Pancreas	Selenium -6	Sugar +7
Liver	Oxygen -7	Hydrogen +6
Adrenal Gland	Iodine -8	Calcium +5
Spleen	Copper -9	Phosphorus +4
Gallbladder	Magnesium -10	Mercury +3
Colon	Fluorine -11	Bismuth +2
Gender F or M	Boron -12	Molybdenum +1

Corrected for Sugar

(*write to me directly if you are scared or need help or want to chat or argue… grove@sent.com Sari Grove…My husband Joseph Grove helps me in everything I do, but if you send me pictures or emails I don't share that with him…I often lose or delete things people send me so I don't have your personal information in my computer…so don't rely on me to store your pictures or anything…I am just here to help…)

Just to compare with a normal Mammogram picture, here is one from my own Mammogram CD…If you have your CD, the file is called the DICOM file there…Open it until you get to black looking slide pictures…Those are your pictures… http://www.dicomlibrary.com/ This service Dicom Library will allow you to anonymously upload your pictures & view them immediately for free online…Anyways,

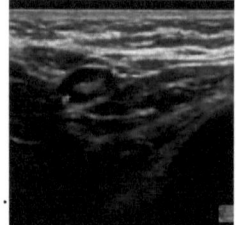

here is one…

You cannot really see very much!

Compare that to my DIY Thermogram process images…You can see both size & chemistry in COLOUR! You can take the photos yourself with no squashing or other people touching you…You can do this every day to see how certain foods or supplements affect size & chemistry…

Blue=Lead(like from alcohol or potatoes or Vitamin A things-antagonize with Vitamin D3 or Ginger root tea)

Light Pink around the Blue=Iron(like from chicken-antagonize with Manganese like Mugwort, Moxa, Moxibustion, bloodroot, or nuts or just Manganese pills)

Almost white around that pink=Aluminum(like cholesterol from eggs type of things-antagonize with Titaniums like Frankincense topically or orally)

The peachy colour around that is Hydrogen=like from water(necrosis is too much Hydrogen not enough Oxygen-hence apricot kernels because they are Oxygen rich)

Yellow is calcium=from Milk(antagonize with Iodines like Iodoral daily 12.5 mg)

Green=Normal flesh

Dark spots=can be Phosphorus(dangerous)(antagonize with a Copper like Licorice root which chases away estrogen Phosphorus fast)

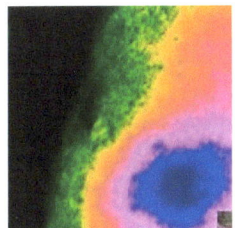

edited at fotoflexer.com

Here is how my picture looks as edited in iPhoto(below)...Here the shiny reflective area is Iron...The foggy grey stuff is Hydrogen...The Blue is Aluminum(cholesterol)...The green is normal tissue...Dark Spots are Phosphorus(which is actually dangerous-antagonize with Licorice root a great Copper that is anti-estrogenic...)How to edit in iPhoto instructions are here...

NOTE:in iPhoto I can see Cholesterol(aluminum) very well-it shows up BLUE...

In iPhoto, if there is a lot of Phosphorus, it shows up as PURPLE...

These two are important to see & do not come up very well in the Fotoflexer.com picture edits...(Sorry! Macintosh discontinued the iPhoto program so I cannot do this for you easily anymore...)If you want me to edit a picture for you in iPhoto(or in Fotoflexer.com) please send me a pic to grove@sent.com & I will do my best to do it quickly...Plus I will probably tell you what I think is there to help...

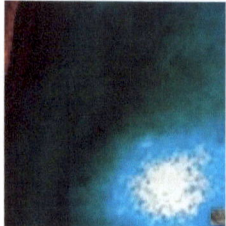

iphoto edit

Note: You can see stuff in other parts of your body too!

When my husband & I were both sick, we wanted to see if it was maybe pneumonia…

I took a picture close-up of Joseph's lung from the back, & I also did a selfie of my own lung taken from my back…(just hold the camera sort of where you think your lung is at your back area)…

I uploaded & edited the photos & compared them to a study that has close u pictures of mouse lungs who had pneumonia…I could see the grey foggy cloudy patches in the lungs of the mice with pneumonia…(grey foggy cloudy patches indicate Hydrogen if you edit in iPhoto…In Fotoflexer, Hydrogen comes out a peachy colour)…

When I looked at our pictures I could also see the same cloudy grey foggy patches…

We did indeed both have pneumonia!

This was important because we stepped up our home treatments…

1000 mg garlic pills(Kyolic), Cayenne pepper in everything including coffee tea & soup…

I also did a 9 minute session at an intermediate(stronger than normal) grade machine at a sun tanning salon…This was key & $25 dollars later,(I also paid for & used the lotion they sell…)my lungs were actually clear…(In winter, a suntanning bed can really boost your system out of a chronic illness, especially in Canada)…

For Joseph, turns out the cayenne pepper in everything was key to his recovery…

A letter I wrote to somebody recently:(with personal stuff removed)

Most lumps or tumours are not made up of cancer cells...

A small fraction may be cancerous, the rest is just Calcium & iron...

A benign lump is calcium Oxalate(oxalate means iron)...

a malignant lump is Calcium phosphate...

So the difference between the two is the Phosphorus...

To prevent & reverse the spread of Phosphorus you use Coppers...Anything in the Copper family will antagonize the Phosphorus & reverse...

Its called Phenotypic reversion when cancer cells return back to normal cells...

I used Licorice root for my Copper because it absorbs well...Tincture, tea, capsules, the raw herb, the herb boiled, even a strong syrup thing...

Ginkgo Biloba is another Copper...

Green tea contains alot of Copper & some people have extracted the catechins from green tea into pills...

Once you have stopped any & all Phosphorus & gotten rid of it, you basically just have a benign lump...

Getting rid of Calcium you need Iodine...Iodoral 12.5 mg daily is fine...The herb Madagascar periwinkle is great too...Poke root too...Kelp too...Vinpocetine is a pill that is also an Iodine-great...eat seaweed & sea vegetables...Fucoidan is a new Iodine...

Iodines shrink the Calcium...

Iron is what makes tumours hard...Anything Manganese softens Iron...Bloodroot is a Manganese...So are nuts...Mugwort (Artemisinin) is a manganese...Manganese pills too...

Other elements are particular to what you eat & drink usually...

If you see alot of Hydrogen then you need Oxygen things...I like apricot kernels for

Oxygen because they are so strong & pretty easy to buy...Tamara st. John grinds them in a coffee grinder them eats them in the morning in unsweetened applesauce...They taste bitter so this is a great way to stick with eating alot of them...

I walk 10 km almost daily...It can take 1-1/2 hours...It used to take 3 hours I was so slow...Walking is almost a full time job...

Vitamin D3 50,000 iu a week is a great booster & helps to dissolve Lead...Lead comes from drinking alcohol usually(shows Blue in the Fotoflexer edited pictures)...(this was a new fact to me too actually-that alcohol contains Lead)...

Green is normal tissue yes...

The rest that is not green is not necessarily Cancer, it's just not exactly what should be there...

What I look for is the Phosphorus...In the iPhoto program Phosphorus shows up as tiny purple ants, or dark spots...

In the Fotoflexer program Phosphorus is harder to see...

It can show up as very dark spots...

I am trying to find a program that could maybe show Phosphorus better, because that is an important one to know about...

Phosphorus is the scary one...

Cholesterol(shows Blue in iPhoto edits, or shows pink in Fotoflexer-usually right after the Blue) responds well to Frankincense/Boswellia...

Things that I am not seeing yet in pictures(but would love to be able to in the future if I can find better editing programs)are:

Sugar(though if I ate sugar by accident- a poppyseed salad dressing was spiked as were the dried cranberries in some innocent looking trail mix- the lump shows increased activity, like more spots on it in pictures)...

Nitrogen(like glutens)

But you can feel things get bigger from glutens…

& most people know to avoid sugars…(though fruit sugars people sneak in often)…

I ordered the Ingrid Naiman book about black salve today…(in Canadian currency cause the dollar is low here, plus shipping, it cost me $75…!)Update: read it!

But I guess if I am going to black salve I've gotta read the black salve Bible on it…"(turns out the Facebook group Black Salve discussion is pretty darn good for learning)…

Resource: http://testingcancer.com/index.html *Kelley Metabolic Centre will mail you tubes for blood & urine samples…You get the samples, mail them back(priority shipping less than 7 days!), & they send you back a full profile that includes Cancer spectrum profiling…It costs less than $500, but if you want to know how you are doing, this might be the way to go…I have not done the cancer profile yet…But I am thinking about it…(update: didn't go for it…Instead spent that money on a topical patch system called Lifewave…)(I'd rather spend on medicines than diagnostics)…*

Question I see often: *What could I do if I have cancer & want to detox & rebalance my biochemistry?*

Answer: (from Sari Grove) Here's a recent list I wrote as a comment somewhere else… If you have any questions about anything, feel free to ask… grove@sent.com "After a year of raw vegetable diet,

10 kilometre walking,

licorice root,

madagascar periwinkle,

mugwort,

vitamin d3 50,000 iu,

lots of oil, apple cider vinegar

, potassium,

Boron,

green tea

, hemp oil,

CBD oil,

hulled hemp seeds,

sesame seeds,

cabbage,

broccoli,

carrots,

green apples,

nuts,

wheatgrass juice,

baking soda,

garlic pills & raw garlic,

apricot kernels,

goji berries,

organic food,

iodoral tablets,

kelp,

poke root,

blue flag iris,

matcha tea,

cold brewed coffee,

gingko biloba,

vinpocetine,

Unda 17(for parasites),

Miror EPF(also for parasites),

black walnut hull,

wormwood,

clove,

(those 3 also for parasites),

Frankincense resin chewed,

Frankincense water,

Boswellia capsules,

Frankincense topically,

Lymph Detox deodorant,

Ginger root boiled,

Epsom Salt baths,

Myrrh oil drops(Opoponax was the species of Myrrh)

magnesium," (I also took Dr. Reckeweg R38, & R39, which gets rid of Ovarian Cysts)…(I also used the Get-ITGirl(get-it girl.com) smoothie powder & Matcha tea powder at the very beginning)(VegaOne Sugar Free Energizer with ginger & turmeric helped at the beginning too!) (Cayenne pepper in everything & ginger root boiled to make tea)…(You can chew Frankincense resin, then spit out the gum later- good medicine!)…I cheated on the raw vegetable diet with fish if I needed proteins…

What about Cancers or Polyps in other parts of the body?

My feeling is that generally speaking with these type of things, the list of things I did would be helpful…It's a systemic thing…Topical salves get rid of lumps & bumps but you really have to detox & rebalance the whole system so nothing comes back & everything is reversed back to normal…The most important ones if you think it's Cancer are:**Licorice Root(for the Copper-alternatively you can get Copper from Ginkgo Biloba & Green Tea), Iodoral or another Iodine but strong & daily…Manganese acts like Bloodroot- you can get Manganese from the herb Mugwort…Boron is very useful in the lower body regions like the Bladder…**

Things I am planning on doing soon…

Bloodroot capsules internally from ZENITH HERBALS…(update: got them & started taking them!)

Black Salve topically on lump to remove it from Zenith herbals…(maybe)(update: still a maybe Nov. 2015)…

Please join the Black Salve Discussion Group on Facebook if you are considering Black Salve or the Bloodroot capsules…You will need them…

Brain Parts	Body Parts	Minus	Plus
Minus	" There are two	female ♀	Male ♂
Plus	sides to every	-	+
12 Brain Part Locations	body part "...	chromosome	chromosome
Frontal Lobe -right / Frontal Lobe left +	Thyroid left Thyroid right	Zinc-1	Lead+12
Motor Cortex- right / Motor Cortex+left	Thymus left Thymus right	manganese-2	Iron+11
Parietal Lobe - right / Parietal Lobe+left	left Lung & Lymph Node right / Lung & Lymph Node	Titanium-3	Aluminum+10
Medulla Oblongata -Top / Medulla Oblongata+bottom	Heart left Heart right	Potassium-4	Aurum+9
Pons -Top / Pons + Bottom	Kidney left Kidney right	Carbon-5	Nitrogen+8
Occipital Lobe- / Occipital Lobe+left	Pancreas left Pancreas right	Selenium-6	Sugar +7
Cerebellum - Right / Cerebellum+left	Liver bottom Liver top	Oxygen-7	Hydrogen+6
Pituitary Gland - Right / Pituitary Gland+left	Adrenal Gland bottom / top Adrenal Gland	Iodine-8	Calcium+5
Globus Palladus-front / Hypothalamus+back	bottom Spleen Spleen top	Copper-9	Phosphorus+4
Broca's Area - front / Wernicke's Area+Back	Gallbladder top / bottom Gallbladder	Magnesium-10	Mercury+3
Temporal Lobe- Right / Pineal Gland+left	Colon bottom Colon top	Fluorine-11	Bismuth+2
Corpus Callosum -front / Cerebral Aqueduct+back	Skene's Gland ♂ / Prostate Gland	Boron-12	Molybdenum+1

copyright GroveCanada2015

24 chromsomes(one extra for the Baker)

Explanation:

"Each body part has two elements that live together as opposites in balance…Disease is an imbalance of these two elements…Find out which body part or corresponding brain part your disease is affecting…Find out if you have an excess or a lack…Lower the correct element if there is excess…Raise the correct element if there is lack…Since they are opposites, by raising one element, you will naturally also lower the other element…It is like a scale or a see-saw…Minus elements detoxify, Plus elements feed…The strongest Minus element is Boron…The strongest Plus element is lead…The numbers indicate how strong an element is…Boron is -12 very strong detoxifier…Lead is +12 very strong feeder…"

Sari Grove

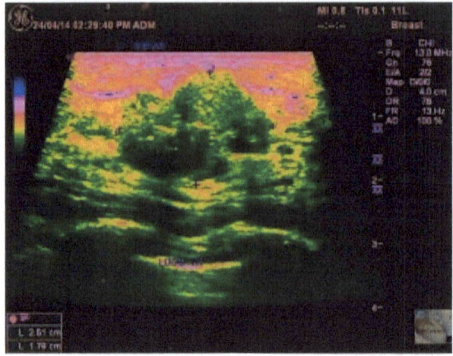

you can do fotoflexer or iphoto edits with ultrasound pictures too

At the end of writing my 3rd book, I discover that Coppers are able to prevent & reverse spread…They don't remove a lump, but can make it revert back to benign…It is called Phenotypic reversion when cancer cells revert back to benign…With my brother's help, I landed on Licorice root as the Copper I would predominantly use…I tracked its effect with my DIY thermogram photo editing-almost daily…Started with St. Francis Licorice root tincture…Once I saw that it was working, my fear about the whole spread thing went away…You can live with a benign lump indefinitely…People forget that…As long as you neuter it, you don't necessarily have to shrink it or take it out-which can be difficult because a benign lump is usually Calcium Oxalate(oxalate means iron) which is almost as hard as a tooth…

Why I had to invent my own imaging program…

…My first & only mammogram tore tissue at the top of both breasts & under the lump…3 months later at my first & only oncologist appt. she said she felt nodes in my non- lump breast…I said yes I know, that was from the mammogram…As a small breasted woman, I have always feared getting up on that table- now I know my fears were warranted…I also had the joy of my pleura being pierced during the core needle biopsy…That means for 2 months when I drank water it went into my lungs…Turns put once again, small breasts plus lump near chest wall can result in accidental piercing called a pneumothorax…This year I tried ultrasound alone(if you try hard enough they let you do this)…So this time they say there are 2 new trails…I say, yes, because you are seeing the trails from the core needle biopsy- they leave 2 straw like trails…So long story short-I was motivated to do my own diagnostic imaging…

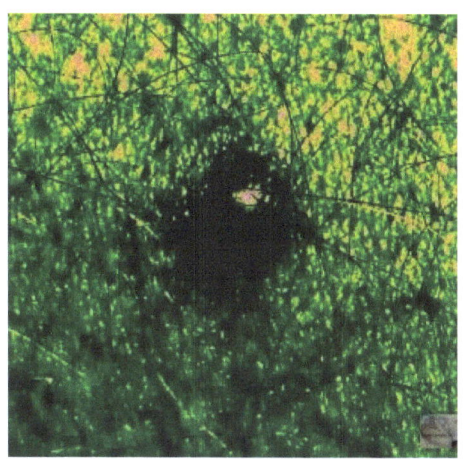

papillomavirus-notice it is dark green(phosphorus signature), whereas the rest of the skin is light green(yellow is calcium)

Alcohol:When I take my pictures & edit them, alcohol comes up as Lead, just like red meat does…It was surprising to me so I researched & found indeed alcohol does have a high Lead content…You can offset that with things like Vitamin D3, Vitamin C, Ginger root tea, Sunshine…The other thing that comes up from alcohol is Hydrogen…You can offset that with Oxygens like Apricot kernels, Goji berries, Milk thistle…Some people burn those things off quickly though, so they can drink…Depends on the person & how active they are…Insomniacs tend to burn off alcohol fast, athletes too…The sugar is another issue…Offset with Lysine, garlic, selenium, pancreatic enzymes…

Note:if you already have Thermogram images, just upload them to Fotoflexer & choose Color Rotate in Effects…(In regular thermograms the red is Lead(blue) on our chart, & the yellow is Iron(light pink)…

If you already have ultrasound images, mammogram images, brain scan images, CT scans, just edit them the same way you would a normal picture, using our steps…)

*If you edit a regular Thermogram picture in Lunapic for malignancy, just SKIP the THERMAL effect step-that has already been done…Also SKIP the ADJUST light levels… Here are the full check for malignancy only instructions…*http://grovecanada.ca/checking-only-for-malignancyphosphorus-after-looking-at-a-lump-or-where-a-lump-was-or-just-checking-under-the-skin-somewhere/

Lungs:

Do you know where exactly in your lungs those nodules were? If you have a digital camera, you could try taking a picture exactly where you think they are…Set to Macro, flash on, about 4-5 inches away…Maybe we could see them? Just a thought…

There is a camera app in the iTunes Store called Camera+ …It turns the iPhone camera into a camera that can be set to Macro, Flash on, & Stabilizer…To take better pictures…Just an idea if you only have an iPhone…

http://grovecanada.ca/so-you-want-to-go-alternative-with-your-cancer-treatment-but-you-dont-know-where-to-start/ If you are starting an Alternative anticancer program & need some guidance, or are already doing one & feel confused, check out my blog post about all that…

(from Sari Grove-& Joseph Grove too)*****I put together a short Kindle book on Amazon, for those who want a copy of these free instructions on Kindle…It is $2.99 American currency)…The book is called DIY Diagnostic Imaging, & contains the short pdf file with just 4 pictures of what to do in Fotoflexer, the written notes on how to just look for malignancy in Lunapic.com, & the so you want to start an alternative anticancer protocol but don't know where to start, blogpost…here is the link http://www.amazon.ca/gp/product/B017HH1RV4?keywords=diy%20diaGnostic%20imaging&qid=1446641370&ref_=sr_1_1&sr=8-1

This post is ONLY the UP CLOSE instructions to check for Phosphorus malignancy…That is ALL it sees, nothing else… http://grovecanada.ca/checking-only-for-malignancyphosphorus-after-looking-at-a-lump-or-where-a-lump-was-or-just-checking-under-the-skin-somewhere/

(here's a free PDF file of the instructions in step by step pictures you can download now…**how to see a lump yourself…**)PDF file 899 kb(small file)

*If you are stuck with these instructions, message me on Facebook (Sari Grove), with your picture & I will edit it for you & walk you through how to again…Or write at grove@sent.com if you don't have Facebook…

- **** asterisk marked comments are all optional, so skim through them…***

http://h.theapp.mobi/diythermogram This is a Free Mobile App that has all these instructions, the video, the short pdf, conveniently in a place you can bookmark on your Mobile Phone & or share with a friend…

***Note: If you are on a laptop, go to the iTunes store & download a Flash browser like Puffin…The free photo editor works on Flash, so you need a Flash browser app to edit your photos there from an iPad…

****Also: The Camera+ App for iPhone has Macro, automatic flash, & Stabilizer- to take better pictures with your iPhone…I usually use my Sony Dsc-T100 point & shoot digital camera set to Macro, Flash on, close up but not so close the flash ruins the picture 3 inches away about…But I have successfully taken photos with an iPad & an iPhone- take your time, good light, close up don't try to get the whole body part, just the place where there is trouble…If there is no lump, you can still see what is happening systemically- very useful for Cancer prevention…You can also take pictures inside your mouth- teeth have problems years before tumours appear- check your mouth now!

*****If you only have an iPhone…Download the Puffin App from the iTunes store…Or any other Flash Browser app you like there…Then when you go to Fotoflexer.com it will work…When you have to move the Hue & Saturation sliders, switch to Fullscreen so the page doesn't move…It is doable…Then exit fullscreen to get the Heat Map & Color Rotate functions…You have to click the More button at the top far right to see them…If your iPhone camera picture is mediocre, download the Camera+ App too…Take your picture with Macro, Stabilizer, (not necessarily flash on because it may be too close & ruin the colours)…You can enhance that picture in the Edit mode if you want it even better before you upload to Fotoflexer…((clarity, sharpen, saturation etc)…

How to do it…(Basic Instructions, again!!!)

Take a picture with your camera set to Macro Flash on about 4 inches away(with iPhone camera set to HDR on, iPad cameras & even pretty crummy cameras WILL work!)…

Too close & the flash will be too strong(so get close, then back off so the Flash doesn't ruin the picture-4-5 inches-take a few shots at different distances)…

Upload to http://www.Fotoflexer.com…

In Basics adjust Hue(all the way to the left, the slider) & Saturation(move this slider

all the way to the right)…

In Effects choose Heat Map…Then choose Color Rotate…

*(after editing in Fotoflexer)Bonus: If you really want to see if there is Phosphorus (malignancy) present, here is an extra step you can take to make sure…Not hard to do…Go to the free photo editor called BeFunky at http://www.Befunky.com…Upload the ALREADY edited picture you edited already in Fotoflexer…The third icon at the far left of the page once you upload is the EDIT button…When you CLICK that button, a bunch of choices come up…The first one to choose is COLOR…When you select that you will see Hue slider, Saturation slider & Temperature slider…MOVE the SATURATION slider all the way to the RIGHT…Click on the checkmark to save that choice…Last step-Choose SHARPEN…Move that SLIDER all the way to the right too! Click the checkmark to save…At the top of the page you can SAVE your picture…The Dark Green spots of Phosphorus will be much more apparent now…

Other editing ideas(non-essential to know/optional):If you want to see just the Phosphorus parts up close(Phosphorus indicates malignancy so it is an important marker, if not the most important) I have a way to see it better…AFTER doing the regular Fotoflexer edit, that that finished edited picture, & save it to your iPhone(sorry this is the way I have done it so far- will try to figure out the online way soon…)
ok…Import the photo into the Camera+ app for iPhone…Choose Edit…In the LAB pro functions…Choose Clarity pro & slide both sliders all the way to the right…Sharpen all the way…Saturation all the way…In Brightness & Contrast- Only slide the Contrast slider all the way to the right…Ok, Done & Save your picture…The dark green spots of Phosphorus will be much easier to see & track…(will add when I find another way to do this)…

Apologies:My brother is at times a bit dyslexic, & when I am around him, sometimes it rubs off…I have reversed Sulphur & Sugar on my Grove Body Part Chart previously, & more recently, discovered a reversal of Aluminum & Iron in my images here…I am so sorry…I do correct mistakes as I find them, but am aware that I may have screwed up your protocols a bit…Please inform me when things are reversed-I am re-editing all 9 manuscripts on Amazon this Christmas season, so this is the time to write to me to tell me new things I may have missed… grove@sent.com or find me on Facebook! Sari Grove p.s. Seasons greetings by the way…If you need help with anything, write…(For those who have been treating themselves for high Iron instead of high Aluminum, rest assured you have not screwed yourself up…Manganese is just a little lighter than Titanium as a medicine, so you just may have under-dosed a bit…Not a fatal mistake, promise!)

Here is an example of a man who went to a strip club to see what it was like…These are two edits of the same photograph…The first is in Fotoflexer, which looks for size & chemistry changes…The second is in LunaPic which looks for (purple) malignancy(foreign creatures)…

This is the same photo, taken of the man, close up of his face…The green area central in the Fotoflexer picture is what the man thought was a "pimple", which had not healed…The photo shows that much more than a pimple occurred after being exposed to the filthy air in the strip club atmosphere, where lap dances are common…The first photo should be all light green if the man had not gone into the strip club at all…This is an example of the type of chemistry your facial skin is exposed to in these adult entertainment clubs…

The Lunapic photo looks for malignancy, or foreign bodies or creatures…They show up as purple…One can see just the beginnings of purple at the bottom edge where the pink ends…So there has been exposure to dangerous foreign parasites…However, for the time being, one would say that the man is relatively cancer free…For now…Let's hope these pictures serve as a warning…Brothels, strip clubs, lap dance parlours, adult entertainment clubs, are rife with disgusting people, odours, drugs, & sexually transmitted diseases…For the amount of money people spend in these places, one should be able to sue for health violations…

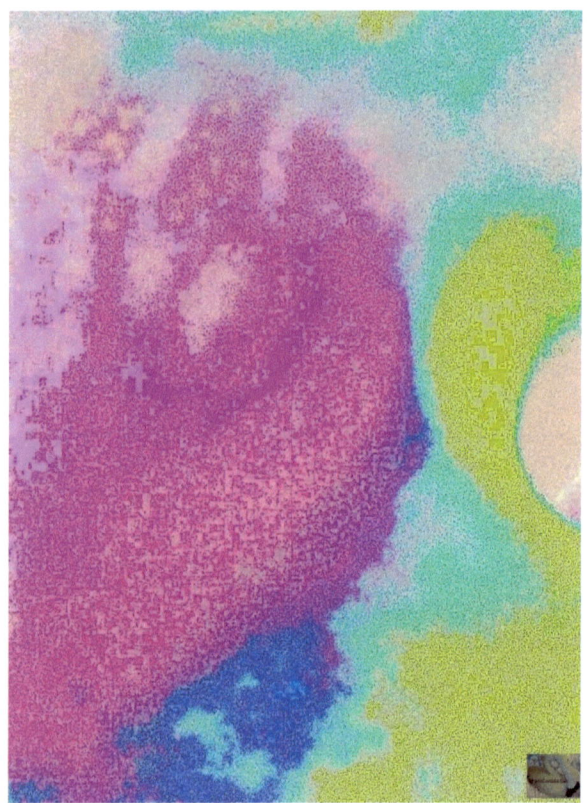

Lunapic

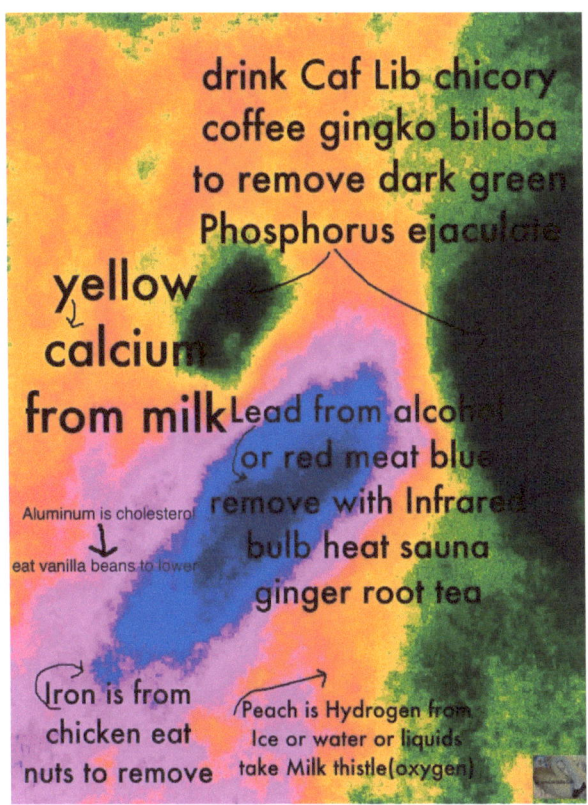

Fotoflexer

Checking only for malignancy(Phosphorus) AFTER looking at a lump or where a lump was or just checking under the skin somewhere...

by Sari - Sunday, November 01, 2015

http://grovecanada.ca/checking-only-for-malignancyphosphorus-after-looking-at-a-lump-or-where-a-lump-was-or-just-checking-under-the-skin-somewhere/

Video shows how to do DIY Diagnostic Imaging in Lunapic to check for malignancy...photo in video taken with iphone 5s camera...

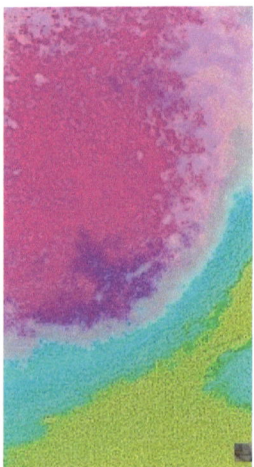

The purple Phosphorus indicates malignancy

After you try the How to see a lump or anything else, like what is going on under your skin systematically, instructions...You may want to take a closer look to see if there is any Phosphorus present...

Phosphorus indicates malignancy...(Use Coppers like licorice root extract, Spirulina, green tea, Cilantro, Yerba Mate, Copper, Plant caffeines, coffee, tea, chromium, St. John's wort, wheatgrass, barley grass, to clear that up...

So...if you want to do the intense checking yourself...Here is how to do ONLY that...

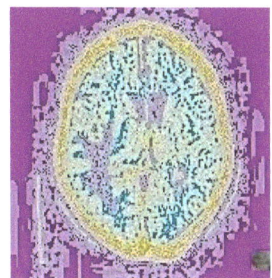

picture shows breast cancer metastasis to brain, edited from CT scan, purple areas indicate malignancy (Phosphorus)...

This is just to see Phosphorus only...nothing else...

Using LunaPic http://www.lunapic.com

These are the new instructions for that...(for people who don't have the iPhoto program...but also, it seems to see it better than iPhoto a bit actually)...

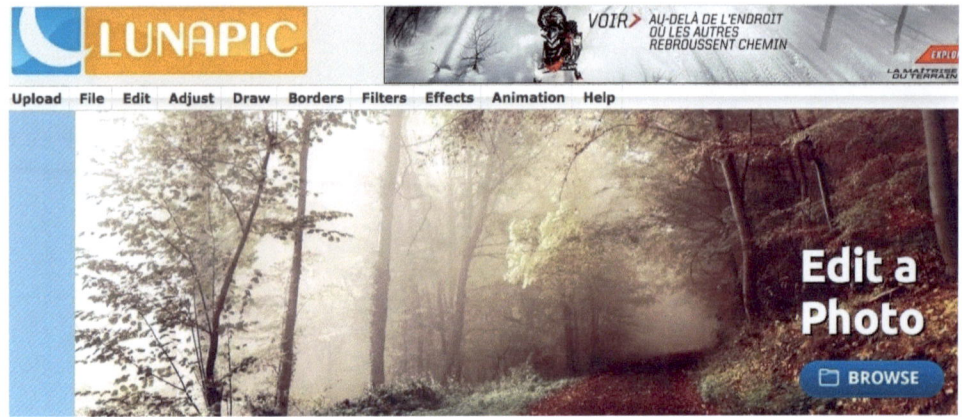

Go to Lunapic.com & Browse for your picture

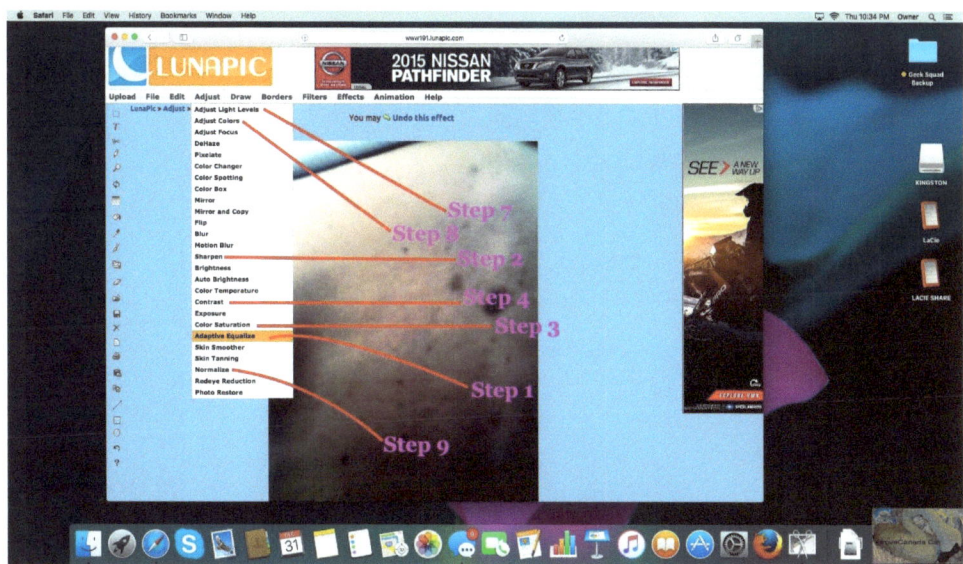

In ADJUST, Adaptive equalize, then Sharpen(all the way to right), then Color Saturation(slider all the way to 100), then Contrast(5 times /click + sign 5 times)…don't forget to hit Apply on each one! (Note:You have to do step 5 & 6, before you can do steps 7 & 8)…

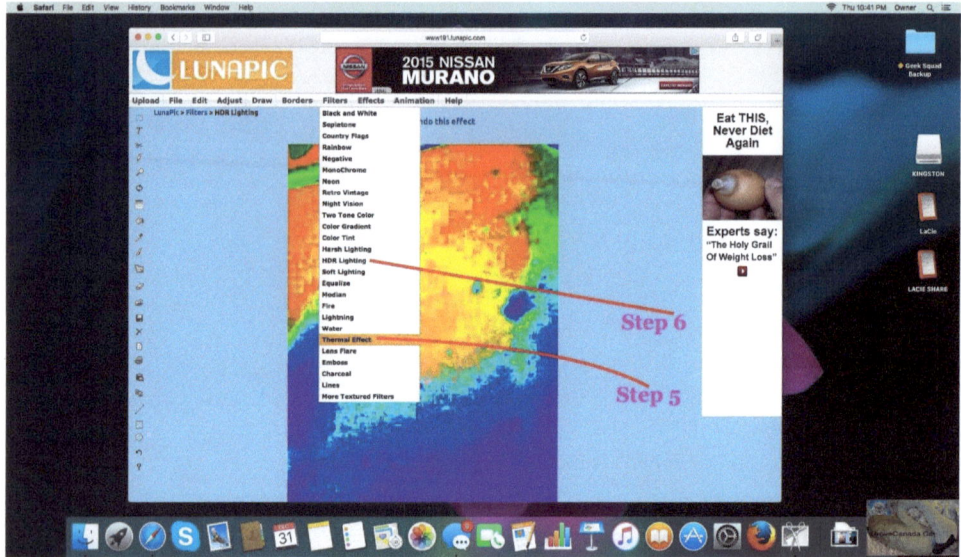

In FILTERS choose Thermal Effect, then HDR Lighting(steps 5 & 6)

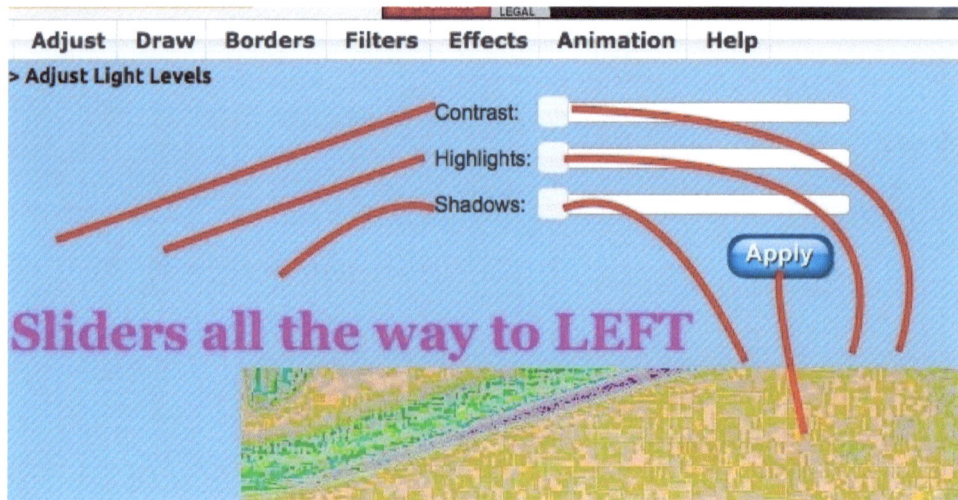

In Adjust, Adjust light levels, slide all 3 sliders to the LEFT then Apply! (Step 7)

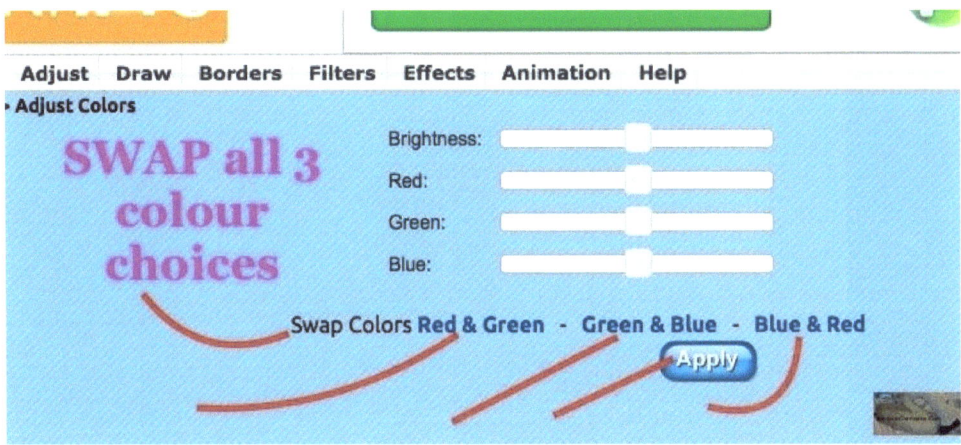

SWAP all 3 colour choices in Adjust Colors(In ADJUST)…then APPLY (Step 8)

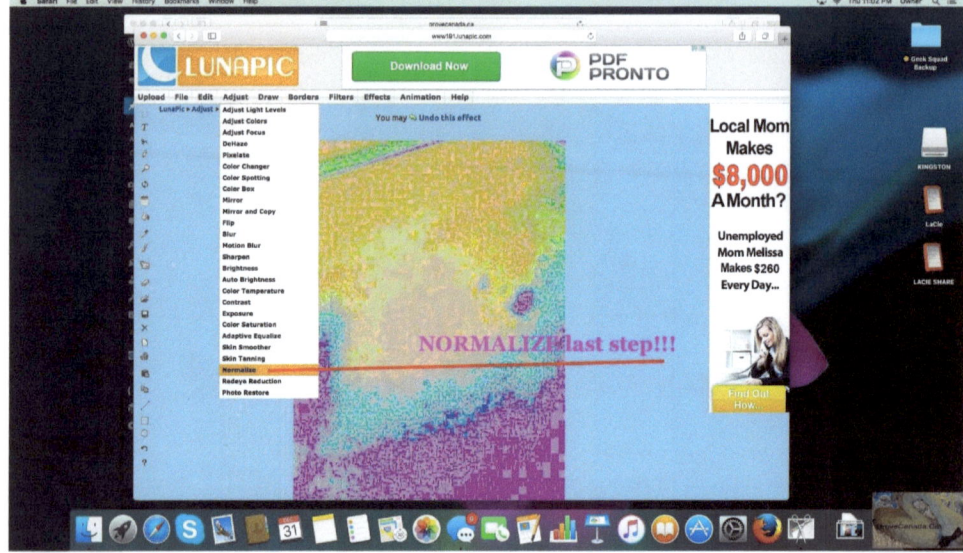

Last step! In ADJUST choose NORMALIZE…Purple indicates presence of Phosphorus
Malignancy…

Ok, here goes…It is not hard, just step by step slow…(wait till each
page loads before going to next step…)
****In Lunapic.com http://www.lunapic.com

IF YOU REALLY WANT TO CHECK
FOR PHOSPHORUS(malignancy) up close:

Follow these steps…

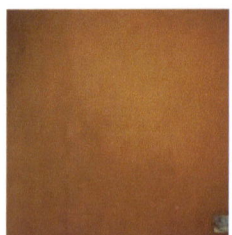

Browse, Upload

Browse(for picture), Upload…

In Adjust:
click adaptive equalize, apply

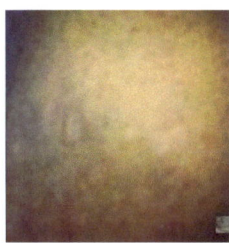

Adaptive Equalize, Apply(in ADJUST)

click sharpen, slider all the way to right(100%), apply
click color saturation, slider all the way to right, apply
contrast-5x (click this 5 times slowly, wait in between for it to fully
load), apply
IN Filters:
thermal effect, apply
HDR lighting, apply
back In Adjust:
adjust light levels—contrast slider to left,

highlights slider to left,
shadows sliders to left

 (all down(to left)), apply
adjust colors:
click the swap red green button
click swap green blue button
click swap blue red button,apply
Normalize, apply,

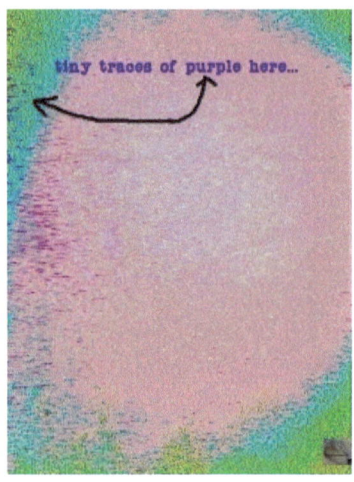

this lump is pretty much all clear of purple

DONE! (in this edit in Lunapic you are looking for purple Phosphorus only...Any purple is Phosphorus, malignancy...(Treat with Coppers like licorice root tincture/extract)

Sari

Video notes for video below:This person has been eating alot of yogurt, kefir, cottage cheese, products & that is showing up temporarily as purple Phosphorus...True malignancy purple has an organic irregular cell shaped creature ant look to it...(Salmonella Typhi bacteria are what we are looking for when we say malignancy...They have a Phosphorus visual signature because that is their favorite food...)

Also note:Before your period your natural body Phosphorus levels rise-don't freak out...Try to take your pictures after your period when things look better so you don't scare yourself!

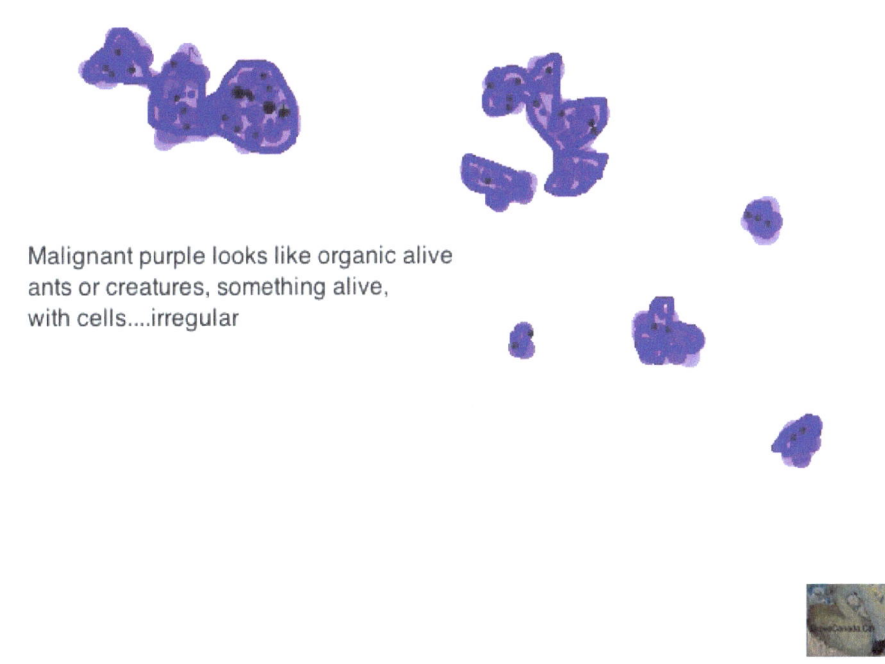

Malignant purple looks like organic alive
ants or creatures, something alive,
with cells....irregular

Malignant Purple looks like creatures

In the Video, go to Settings(its a little circle in the bottom right hand corner of the video frame, & TURN ON ANNOTATIONS…I have written some messages on the video that are important…)

(If you edit a regular Thermogram picture that you already have, in Lunapic for malignancy, just SKIP the THERMAL effect step-that has already been done…Also SKIP the ADJUST light levels…)

Reminder:Salmonella typhi bacteria show up as Phosphorus purple but they also like to eat Phosphorus purple...In your check for malignancy picture, the salmonella typhi bacteria will look odd shaped, organic, alive, like ants-they will be irregular...Phosphorus that you have just eaten will show up as flat purple, regular, abstract, not alive looking, no cells, in a constrained area...Lowering your overall Phosphorus levels gets rid of salmonella typhi bacteria, malignancy, but don't freak out if you eat cottage cheese one day or yogurt & your Phosphorus levels show as being really alot...This is probably only temporary...Wait a day, two days, three days, & take another picture...try not to scare yourself...

Differentiating Malignancy from Cottage cheese, yoghurt, kefir, or natural body Phosphorus visual signatures...

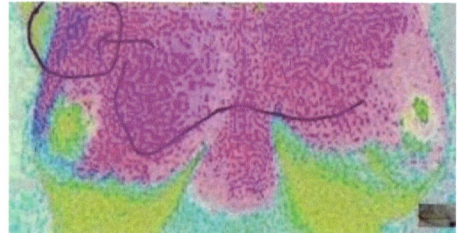

Inflammatory Breast Cancer-Purple at far left(arrow) is irregular, notice"wormy" texture on chest, some purple tones there too...

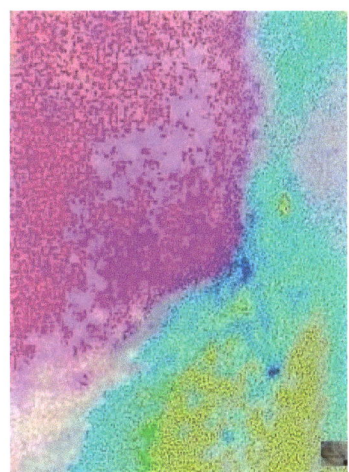

Lunapic edit (still from first video of this post)this person has been drinking soy milk, cow milk, eating cheese, & taking Chaste tree, wild yams, & soy isoflavones

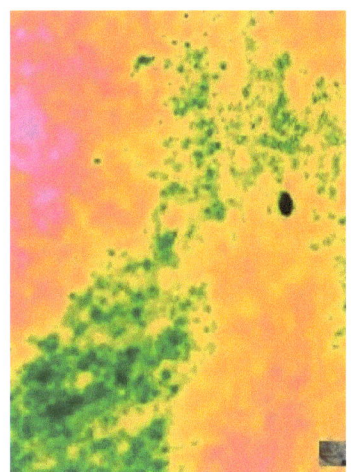

same picture in fotoflexer edit

Question: How much licorice root did you take?

Answer:

I didn't have a system…

For how much I would take…

I just took pictures every day, to see if the Phosphorus was gone…

I dosed according to how I felt, how it made me feel, how much money I wanted to spend that week, how afraid I was…

If you can keep track of it once in a while in pictures, it will help you to know how you are doing…

What I did find was that when you order a mega-bottle of extract, you get way too much alcohol & not a whole lot of extract…

My husband says that is normal-they get sloppy & sell you dilute stuff…

So I went back to the small bottles…

Also layered in tea, capsules, the herb simmered on stove then drink liquid, also just swallowed herb raw…

I was trying to make it all cheaper…

Possibly I should not have done that…

The cheaper you spend maybe the less strong it is…

The extract really made me feel the burn…

I did get that feeling from the other stuff but not as much…

There are other things in the same category (Copper) that give you a buzz too…

Gingko biloba, copper supplements, spirulina, chlorella, coffee, tea, matcha, chromium, boron, yerba mate, plant caffeines, really anything caffeinated(energy drinks), st. john's wort…cocaine(no I did not do this, but it is a copper, as is crack cocaine), gotu kola, kola nut, um…I am probably repeating myself, I forget sometimes how many times I have said the same thing…

http://www.amazon.com/Diagnostic-Imaging-Grove-Health-Science-ebook/dp/B017HH1RV4/ref=sr_1_1?ie=UTF8&qid=1446676018&sr=8-1&keywords=diy+diagnostic+imaging

I stuck what we did into a short Kindle book for the time being…It probably needs to be edited, but I put it up fast(literally stuck it together on my iphone from blog posts)…Just in case people need this now…

With the Saint Francis Licorice root extract I took 4 dropperfuls a day to start…

I basically gulped the whole bottle in 3 days…

Hence me trying to find a cheaper way…

I think ideally, people might just stick with that if they can…

I like your 3 times a day idea…

That would be faster…

I took some sort of licorice root for a year…(9 capsules of licorice root daily)

After a year, I started to overdose…

You get a panicky emotion if you overdose…

That is when you know you are overdosing...

If it gets really bad you have to actually ADD back a Phosphorus, like Kefir(liquid yogurt)...It is dangerous to do that, but the panic emotion is tough...It is fun to drink Kefir though after a year of no dairy allowed!

Sari

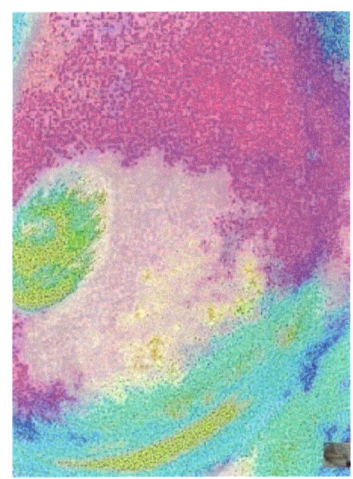

see the purple in the top right hand corner?

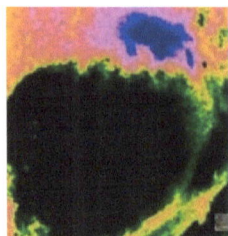

same subject but this edited in fotoflexer the green spots at top right

Note:Malignancy, Phosphorus, Salmonella Typhi bacterium, & Yogurt or other Phosphorus foods, will all show up as purple(In the Lunapic edit)…It is definitely a sign that your Phosophorus levels are too high, but don't freak out-it may just be excessive yogurt eating…Until we make this process even more specific, please be aware that it is not perfect…Sorry…This takes time to figure out & we need the right people & the right picture to be able to discern things…

How to differentiate between an active malignancy or just temporary presence of Phosphorus due to eating cottage cheese, cheese, yogurt, Kefir, milk, soy, tofu or other Phosphorus items…

First of all- if you have not eaten any Phosphorus containing foods or supplements(probiotics, 5HTP tryptophan, valerian root, GABA, Kav Kava, may all show up as Phosphorus), & your picture shows purple, then your purple is probably indicating malignancy…

If you have been eating any Phosphorus foods or supplements, then the purple in your picture may be temporary food Phosphorus…Stop eating those foods or supplements for 3 days then take another picture…If the purple clears up, it was nothing to worry about…

photo in video taken with camera+ app from itunes store with lens reversed, macro, stabilizer, flash on…